We would like to thank the many teachers and trainee teachers who trialled and helped to develop practical ideas in this book. We are also grateful to the staff, pupils and parents of Mountfields Lodge Primary School in Loughborough and Hamilton College in Leicester for allowing us to take photographs in their schools.

Contents

Preface

Helping children lead healthy, active lifestyles has become increasingly important as we have learned more about the ill-health consequences of sedentary living, as well as the current health status and low activity levels of a significant proportion of young people. In response to such concerns, school curricula around the world are placing increased emphasis on promoting healthy, active lifestyles. This book will help you and your school create such an emphasis and support you in your efforts to promote active lifestyles among young people.

More specifically, the book is designed to help you make a positive difference to your pupils' health, well-being and quality of life by equipping them with the knowledge, skills, understanding, competence and confidence to engage in a physically active lifestyle. It will also help schools address this important element of the curriculum in a planned, progressive manner that is accessible to all pupils.

Promoting Active Lifestyles in Schools is intended for all persons involved in promoting healthy, active lifestyles in schools: primary school teachers; secondary school teachers; personal, social, health and economic education coordinators; healthy-school coordinators; health, physical activity, physical education and sport coordinators in schools, local authorities and communities; health, physical activity, physical education and school sport consultants, advisers and providers of professional development; and primary and secondary school teacher educators.

Scope

In terms of breadth, the book addresses curriculum requirements (in both physical education and other subjects); whole-school and cross-curricular recommendations and expectations; extracurricular opportunities; and links with parents and physical activity providers in the community. It includes a diverse range of activities that can be undertaken both within and beyond school buildings. This range accommodates schools that can deliver lessons (in physical education and other subjects) in the surrounding environment beyond the classroom. In addition, it offers best-practice case studies to help you visualise and conceptualise how to implement practices that promote activity. Throughout, the book's content is based on evidence and informed by research drawn from the findings of studies conducted by the authors and eminent researchers around the world.

Content Overview

Promoting Active Lifestyles in Schools contains a mixture of practical ideas and activities, alongside explanations based on current thinking and evidence. It is structured in three parts. Part I explains the importance of promoting healthy, active lifestyles in schools and clarifies how schools in general, and physical education in particular, can do so. Part II focuses on how children's health, activity and fitness can be monitored in schools and how this monitoring can help pupils learn the importance of being healthy, active and fit in their everyday lives. Part III addresses how children of all ability levels can be involved in a healthy, active lifestyle, including children with specific health conditions such as asthma, diabetes and obesity. It also presents a range of health-related learning activities for pupils of various ages that are developmentally appropriate, inclusive and progressive.

Specific features of the book include the following:

- Practices based on evidence and informed by research on health-related pedagogies around the world
- Practical learning activities that are tried and tested for helping pupils of all ages lead a healthy, active lifestyle

- Clear explanations of the current thinking and evidence underpinning the practical ideas and activities
- Developmentally appropriate procedures for monitoring children's health, activity and fitness in schools
- Best-practice case studies to help you visualise and conceptualise how the principles outlined in the book can be implemented using real-life practices that promote activity

How to Use the Web Resource

The web resource, found at www.Human Kinetics.com/PromotingActiveLifestyles InSchools, includes a variety of useful materials that you may either print and use as is or adapt to suit your needs. Specifically, you will find the following: a quiz addressing children's health, activity and fitness recommendations; true-or-false statements associated with debunking myths and misconceptions about children's health, activity and fitness; a parent information sheet (An Hour a Day Keeps the Doctor at Bay!); lifestyle case studies; health behaviour questionnaires; physical activity diaries; developmentally appropriate fitness tests; reflective questions; and worksheets for use with pupils of various age groups. These resources exemplify the pedagogical principles recommended in the book and will help you implement activity-promoting practices. The resource also includes a list of web links to help you learn more about the many initiatives and guidelines mentioned in the book.

Promoting Active Lifestyles in Schools will help you and your school promote healthy, active lifestyles in a planned, progressive manner that is accessible to all pupils. These efforts will make a positive difference to the health, well-being and quality of life of your pupils by equipping them with the knowledge, skills, understanding, competence and confidence to engage in physically active lifestyles.

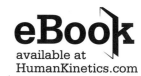

How to Access the Web Resource

Throughout *Promoting Active Lifestyles in Schools*, you will notice previews of supplemental materials that can be found in the web resource. This online content is available to you free of charge when you purchase a new print or electronic version of the book. The web resource offers printable and editable supplemental materials such as worksheets, assessments, information sheets, and more. To access the online content, simply register with the Human Kinetics website. Here's how:

1. Visit www.HumanKinetics.com/Promoting ActiveLifestylesInSchools

2. Click the first edition link next to the corresponding first edition book cover.

3. Click the Sign In link on the left or at the top of the page. If you do not have an account with Human Kinetics, you will be prompted to create one.

4. Once you have registered, if the online product does not appear in the Ancillary Items box at the left, click the Enter Pass Code option in that box. Enter the following pass code exactly as it is printed here, including any capitalization and hyphens: **HARRIS-4CRA-WR**.

5. Click the Submit button to unlock your online product.

6. After you have entered your pass code for the first time, you will never have to enter it again in order to access this online product. Once you have unlocked your product, a link to the product will appear permanently in the menu on the left. All you need to do to access your online content on subsequent visits is sign in to www.HumanKinetics.com/Promoting ActiveLifestylesInSchools and follow the link!

If you need assistance along the way, click the Need Help? button on the book's website.

PART I

Promoting Healthy, Active Lifestyles in UK Schools

Recommendations for Nurturing Healthy, Active Children

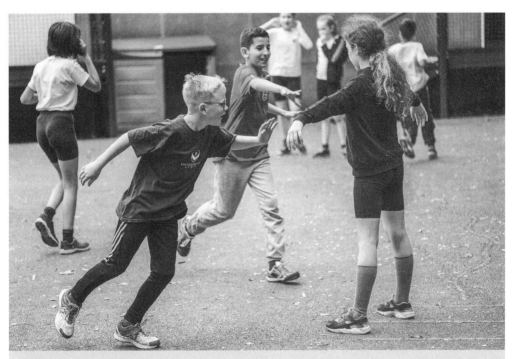

Chapter Objectives

After reading this chapter, you will be able to

- ▶ explain the rationale for promoting physical activity among all children and young people;
- ▶ understand the role of schools and curriculum physical education in promoting healthy, active lifestyles;
- ▶ describe worldwide and UK recommendations on physical activity for health for children and young people;
- ▶ identify reasons for the shift from exercise recommendations and fitness test batteries to holistic physical-activity guidelines and education programmes that promote activity and fitness; and
- ▶ recognise gaps in children's and young people's knowledge and understanding of health, fitness and physical activity that may hinder the promotion of healthy, active lifestyles.

Schools provide obvious venues for health promotion, and physical education (PE) clearly has a role to play in promoting active lifestyles. However, it is important to reflect critically on how best to fulfil these roles in order to achieve positive health outcomes for all children and young people. To start with, we need to know how active children should be and how best to implement recommendations about activity for health in the school setting. We must also identify and address common gaps in children's knowledge and understanding of health, fitness and physical activity in order to increase their uptake of healthy, active lifestyles. With these concerns in mind, this chapter brings you up to date on the growing evidence base that underpins the promotion of physical activity among children and young people.

Benefits of Regular Physical Activity

A review of worldwide literature provides a strong rationale for promoting healthy, active lifestyles among children (Biddle & Asare, 2011; Department of Health, Department of Health, Social Sciences and Public Safety, Scottish Government, & Welsh Government (2011); Donnelly et al., 2016; Janssen & LeBlanc, 2010; National Institute for Health and Care Excellence [NICE], 2008a, 2008b, 2009, 2015b; Physical Activity Guidelines Advisory Committee, 2008; Public Health England, 2014a, 2014b, 2015). In particular, such a review finds evidence not only that physical activity benefits the health of young people but also that many children are relatively inactive and that they generally become less active as they get older. This finding is especially concerning in light of **hypokinetic** conditions (i.e., those related to inactivity) such as **obesity**. Furthermore, a thorough literature review identifies patterns in health-related behaviours and finds that many of these behaviours are acquired and established during childhood and adolescence.

Evidence shows that physical activity provides children with a range of psychological, social and physical benefits (Biddle & Asare, 2011; Department of Health, Department of Health, Social Sciences and Public Safety, Scottish Government, & Welsh Government, 2011; Donnelly et al., 2016; Janssen & LeBlanc, 2010; NICE, 2008a, 2008b, 2009, 2015b; Physical Activity Guidelines Advisory Committee, 2008; Public Health England, 2014a, 2014b, 2015; Stensel, Gorely, & Biddle, 2008). For example, research finds that increased physical activity provides small but significant benefits in reducing body fat and can play a role in obesity treatment for young people when combined with appropriate dietary modification. Research has also found a beneficial association between physical activity and a range of metabolic factors, such as hypertension (high blood pressure), insulin resistance and lipid and lipoprotein concentrations. In addition, weight-bearing and strength-enhancing physical activity can promote skeletal health in young people. Regular physical activity also reduces risk factors for **chronic conditions** (such as heart disease) and, if maintained into adulthood, reduces the risk of **morbidity** and mortality from various diseases (e.g., cardiovascular disease, diabetes, cancer).

These physical health benefits are particularly important given the increasing rates of obesity among children and the fact that **cardiovascular disease** has its origins in childhood. Childhood obesity is a global issue, as evidenced by a report from the World Health Organisation (WHO, 2016) indicating that the number of **overweight** or obese infants and young children (aged 0 through 5 years) increased from 32 million in 1990 to 42 million in 2013. In England, obesity figures increased from 11 percent of boys and 12 percent of girls aged 2 through 15 in 1995 to 18 percent and 19 percent in 2005. The levels have been slightly lower since then—for example, 16 percent for boys and 15 percent for girls in 2013 (Health and Social Care Information Centre [HSCIC], 2015).

In terms of psychological and social benefits, physical activity that is appropriately structured and delivered can help young people feel better about themselves and reduce symptoms of anxiety and depression (Biddle & Asare, 2011). It can also result in increased self-confidence and self-worth, particularly in disadvantaged groups, such as those with learning or behavioural difficulties and those with initially low self-esteem. Appropriate physical activity can also improve young people's social skills, such as their ability to relate to others, as well as their sense of fair play and justice.

These psychological and social health benefits of physical activity take on increased importance in light of the global prevalence (about 20 percent) of mental health disorders among children and adolescents (WHO, 2005). This concern holds particularly true in the United Kingdom (Tymms et al., 2016) which ranked last on children's well-being among 21 of the world's richest countries in 2007, 16th among 29 in 2013 and 20th out of 35 of the richest countries in 2016 (United Nations Children's Fund, 2007, 2013, 2016). The psychological and social benefits only occur, however, if experiences of physical activity, physical education and sport are positive and explicitly planned and structured to produce particular outcomes. This type of structure is more likely to be used when the efforts are facilitated by well-qualified professionals.

Some research also indicates benefits of physical activity for young people's academic or cognitive performance. Specifically, some studies report weak but positive associations between physical activity (as well as physical fitness) and academic achievement and between fitness and elements of cognitive function (Keeley & Fox, 2009). Other research has indicated a positive effect of activity on cognitive outcomes and academic achievement, with the greatest effect coming from aerobic exercise (Fedewa & Ahn, 2011).

Evidence is also mounting that children benefit from physical fitness. For example, physical fitness is related to a healthy **cardiovascular disease (CVD) risk profile** and to healthy levels of body fatness in children and adolescents; it may also exert a positive influence on psychological health and cognitive performance (Janssen & LeBlanc, 2010). In addition, findings from large-scale studies have suggested that high physical fitness during adolescence and young adulthood is related to a healthy risk-factor profile later in life (Janssen & LeBlanc; Twisk, Kemper, & Van Mechelen, 2002).

Having said all this, the health benefits of physical activity and physical fitness for children are not as well established as they are for adults. In addition, the associations between, on one hand, physical activity and physical fitness and, on the other hand, some health benefits for children appear to be only small or relatively weak. These gaps may result from the following factors:

- We lack a sufficient number of large-scale, longitudinal studies conducted on children, and such studies must contend with difficulties in measuring children's health, fitness and activity.

- Children tend not to engage in sustained vigorous activity or exercise training, which have been the foci of many studies.

- Because children's health cannot be measured by mortality statistics, researchers have relied on CVD risk factors, which represent a relatively crude indicator of cardiovascular health.

- Children's habits associated with a physically inactive lifestyle may have had insufficient time to negatively influence CVD risk factors.

- It may be that an insufficient number of children have been inactive for negative health consequences to be evident.

Nevertheless, a strong rationale exists for promoting physical activity among all children and young people. This rationale is based on the strengthening relationship between physical activity (and physical fitness) and health in children, the fact that CVD has its origins in childhood, and the increasing rates of inactivity-related or hypokinetic health conditions (e.g., obesity) among children.

Risks of Inactivity

Many children are relatively inactive. The World Health Organisation's Health Behaviour in School-aged Children (HBSC) survey reported that less than half of young people met the physical activity recommendation of one hour or more of at-least moderate activity each day (Currie et al., 2008). Even worse, in the United Kingdom, this guideline is not met by the vast majority of children; indeed, only 20 percent of girls and 23 percent of boys in England are at least moderately active for one hour or more on a daily basis (HSCIC, 2016). This pattern of boys being proportionally more active than girls holds true across all countries and all age groups (Organisation for Economic Co-operation and Development [OECD], 2013).

In recent years, physical activity levels have dropped among children and young people; moreover, physical activity tends to decline during adolescence. The Health Survey for England 2015 (HSCIC, 2016) identified decreases between 2008 and 2015 in the proportion of both girls and boys who met health guidelines for physical activity. The decrease was more marked in the oldest age group. Also, time spent being sedentary both during the week and at weekends increased with age (HSCIC, 2016). Having said this, the Health Survey for England excludes school-based activities which clearly form a key source of both sedentary and active behaviours.

Similar patterns have been found among children and young people both in other countries in the United Kingdom—in the Welsh Health Survey 2016 (Welsh Government, 2017), the Scottish Health Survey 2015 (Scottish Government, 2016) and the Young People and Sport in Northern Ireland survey (2016)—and around the world (OECD, 2013). To add to the complexity of the situation, national surveys from all UK countries and international data point to differences in physical activity participation associated with a range of additional variables, such as geographical region, urban or rural location, culture, religion, and special needs and disabilities.

Patterns of health-related behaviours are often acquired and established during childhood and adolescence. For example, physical activity tracks into adulthood (Twisk, Kemper, & Van Mechelen, 2000) and up to 79 percent of children in England who are obese in their teens are likely to remain obese as adults (NICE, 2015; Telema, 2009).

Schools' Effectiveness in Promoting Active Lifestyles

Schools provide an important avenue through which to promote healthy, active lifestyles among children because they

- reach the vast majority of children and adolescents,
- influence children's behaviour for 40 percent or more of their waking time,
- can improve the health of young people by providing programmes and services that promote enjoyable physical activity delivered by professionals and
- can influence not only young people but also their families.

Even so, schools' effectiveness in addressing societal health problems has been questioned for a number of reasons (Gard & Pluim, 2014; St. Leger, 2004; Thomas, 2004). First, school influence does not extend to certain factors that affect young people's health, such as genetics, environment and family modelling. Second,

even as schools are increasingly asked to address public health concerns (e.g., poor nutritional behaviours, unwanted pregnancies, tobacco use), they themselves are grappling with issues such as insufficient training, financial constraints and competing elements in a finite curriculum. Third, some argue that the core business of schools is not to reduce health problems but to focus on educational outcomes (Gard & Pluim, 2014; St. Leger, 2004; Thomas, 2004). Whilst these factors undoubtedly limit schools' effectiveness in addressing societal health problems, they should not stop schools from contributing what they can to health education and promotion among children.

Within this broader context, the promotion of active lifestyles remains a widely accepted goal of school physical education, both in the United Kingdom and across the world (Australian Curriculum and Reporting Authority, 2011; Department for Education, 2013). One reason for this focus lies in the fact that physical educators (along with some teachers of other curriculum subjects) possess appropriate knowledge and expertise. In addition, PE contributes to a broad and balanced curriculum that promotes pupils' spiritual, cultural, mental and physical development. Physical education can also raise awareness, develop knowledge and understanding and enhance positive attitudes in young people with respect to health and physical activity. Indeed, school-based physical activity and physical education programmes (in addition to other aspects of the curriculum) have been shown over the years to promote knowledge and understanding of physical activity, positive attitudes towards PE and physical activity, increased activity and fitness levels and healthy dietary behaviours (as exemplified in reviews by Cale & Harris, 2005, 2006; De Meester, van Lenthe, Spittaels, Lien, & De Bourdeauhuij, 2009; Demetriou & Honer, 2012; Dobbins, De Corby, Robeson, Husson, & Tirilis, 2009; Dobbins, Husson, De Corby, & La Rocca, 2013; Kriemler et al., 2011; Stone, McKenzie, Welk, & Booth, 1998; and van Sluijs, McMinn, & Griffin, 2007).

Health-Related Recommendations for Children

Whilst this book focuses on promoting active lifestyles, the work of doing so must be seen in the broader context of schools' role in encourag-

ROUTE 2 GOOD HEALTH: PROMOTING HEALTHY BEHAVIOURS IN SCHOOLS

One secondary school implemented a whole-school initiative to promote healthy behaviours among its pupils. In particular, the school governors and staff were keen to address childhood obesity as they were aware of an increase in childhood and adult obesity in their geographical area and considered it an issue in their school. As a consequence, the health behaviours targeted were healthy eating, healthy drinking and activity.

The initiative, named Route 2 Good Health, was introduced during assemblies for pupils in years 7 and 8 (i.e., 11- to 13-year-olds) at the beginning of the school year. It was also incorporated into the school's personal, social, health and economic (PSHE) education programme in the form of specific lessons at the start of each school term for years 7 and 8. Parents were informed of the initiative by means of a leaflet taken home by pupils and through information provided on the school's website. Parents were asked to support the initiative by encouraging their children to make healthy food, drink and activity choices (e.g., eating fruits and vegetables and walking or cycling to school).

Discussion points: What possible objections might parents raise to this sort of initiative? How would you deal with parents who took offense at the implication that they were not providing healthy food and drink to their child?

As part of the initiative, each pupil in years 7 and 8 was given a Route 2 Good Health booklet outlining the benefits of healthy eating and drinking and of being active. These benefits were also discussed in the Route 2 Good Health lessons in the PSHE programme, as were the consequences of *not* eating and drinking healthily and of being inactive. The booklet prompted pupils to reflect on their current eating, drinking and activity habits and to consider ways of improving these health behaviours. Planned improvements were recorded in the form of short-term, medium-term and long-term targets.

Discussion point: What are some examples of possible planned improvements in children's eating, drinking and activity habits?

The booklet also included pages on which to record eating, drinking and activity behaviours both in and out of school. Positive health behaviours demonstrated in school—for example, consuming or purchasing healthy meals and drinks at lunchtime and participating in extracurricular physical activity sessions—were rewarded with a stamp in the booklet from canteen staff and teachers. Pupils with the most stamps at the end of each school term received prizes at assemblies. These prizes included vouchers to spend at sport shops or local leisure centres.

Discussion points: Do you think it appropriate to offer extrinsic rewards to motivate children to adopt healthy behaviours? Why, or why not? If they are used, what intrinsic rewards might be offered?

Teachers reported that the pupils generally welcomed the initiative, and there was an increase both in healthy food and drink choices and in participation in extracurricular activity sessions. In addition, pupils gave positive reports on the initiative in school council meetings. Accordingly, a one-year review of the initiative concluded that it had improved the health behaviours of many pupils. Recommendations for the future included recording and rewarding health behaviours performed outside of school and involving parents in confirming or 'stamping' these behaviours.

Discussion points: What are the possible benefits and limitations of increasing parental involvement in the programme? What actions might be taken to help sustain the programme?

ing young people to engage in lifestyles that are healthy overall. Recommendations related to physical activity and diet generally include being active on a daily basis, eating plenty of fruits and vegetables and drinking water instead of fizzy drinks. For example, the Department of Health's 2009 Change4Life campaign helps families and individuals make small, sustainable improvements to their diet, activity levels and alcohol consumption levels. Using the slogan 'eat well, move

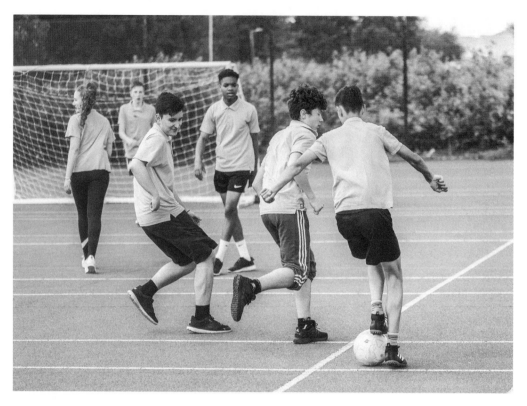

PE programmes and educators can influence and promote healthy levels of physical activity not just in the classroom but for a child's lifetime.

more, live longer', the programme recommends adopting the following six health behaviours:

1. Eating five portions in total of fruits and vegetables each day (e.g., by adding fruit to cereal or choosing canned fruit in its own juice rather than in sugary syrup)

2. Reducing salt intake (e.g., swopping crisps, salted nuts and salty snacks for plain rice cakes, chopped fruit, veggie sticks or unsalted nuts; using less sauce or reduced-salt sauce)

3. Cutting back on saturated fat (e.g., choosing oven chips instead of fried chips; grilling or baking instead of frying; reducing or giving up pastries; choosing reduced-fat cheese)

4. Reducing sugar intake (e.g., replacing jams and chocolate spreads with soft fruits; replacing sweet cereals with low-sugar cereals and fruits)

5. Cutting down on alcohol consumption (e.g., drinking only with meals; resisting pressure to 'keep up' with others; doing something different, such as taking a bath or engaging in a new hobby)

6. Leading an active lifestyle (e.g., gardening; walking or cycling to school or work; taking up an active hobby)

Sport Northern Ireland (2009) has mounted a similar social marketing campaign, Activ8, to raise awareness among primary school children about the importance of daily physical activity and a healthy, balanced diet. The programme promotes the following points:

1. Move your body.
2. Be part of a team.
3. Create your own game.
4. Involve your family.
5. Eat well.
6. Go outdoors.
7. Be a leader.
8. Measure your success.

The World Health Organisation (2008) has established a global strategy on diet, physical activity and health in order to combat increases among children in noncommunicable diseases predominantly related to unhealthy diet and physical inactivity. As part of this strategy, schools are encouraged to consider a range of process and output indicators, such as the following:

- Developing and disseminating a school policy to promote healthy eating and increased physical activity
- Gathering baseline information about pupils' awareness of the benefits of healthy eating and physical activity
- Designing and implementing a plan with clear goals related to the school curriculum and environment

Schools are also asked to consider a range of short-term, intermediate and long-term outcome indicators. Examples include the proportion of pupils demonstrating knowledge and understanding of healthy eating habits and the benefits of physical activity (short-term outcome), participating in at least one hour of physical activity per day (intermediate outcome) and being obese (long-term outcome).

Such campaigns communicate important health messages in straightforward language for their respective audiences. However, their ability to bring about positive changes in behaviour is often constrained by the limited funds available for disseminating key messages to target audiences and evaluating a campaign's effects. Whilst campaigns can make important contributions to positive behaviour change, the reality is that they can do only so much, given the challenge and complexity of changing behaviour, especially behaviour that is well established.

Physical Activity Recommendations for Children

Over the years, experts have produced various physical activity recommendations, such as the global recommendations from the WHO (2010) on physical activity for health for 5- to 17-year-olds (as well as recommendations for younger and older age groups). Specifically, the WHO offers the following recommendations for school-age pupils to reduce signs of anxiety and depression and improve cardiorespiratory and muscular fitness, bone health, and cardiovascular and metabolic health markers:

- Children and young people aged 5 to 17 years old should accumulate at least 60 minutes per day of moderate- to vigorous-intensity physical activity.
- Engaging in more than 60 minutes per day of physical activity provides additional health benefits.
- Most daily physical activity should be aerobic.
- Vigorous-intensity activities should be incorporated, including those that strengthen muscle and bone, at least three times per week.

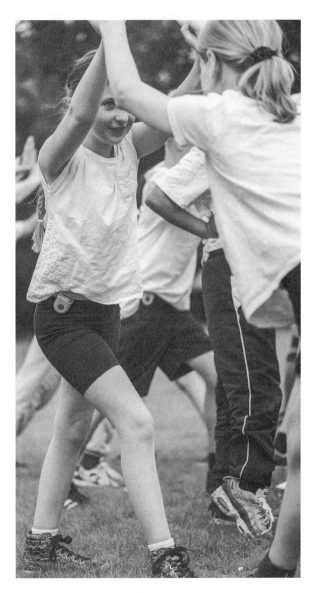

The World Health Organisation provides recommendations for the health and welfare of children around the globe.

For this age group, the WHO proposes that physical activity include play, games, sport, transportation, recreation, and PE or planned exercise in the context of family, school and community activities.

WHO recommendations regarding physical activity for health promote a consistent public health message and are age specific and culturally appropriate. They are also realistic and attainable by the groups for whom they are intended. This quality is enhanced by the emphasis on moderate as well as vigorous physical activity. That is, whilst some vigorous-intensity activity is recommended at least three times per week, physical activity does not have to be strenuous in order to provide benefits. This range of options should make the prospect of participating more appealing for more youngsters. In addition, the message that physical activity can be accumulated over the course of the day makes the recommendations particularly appropriate for younger children, whose activity patterns tend to be sporadic and transitory.

The recommendations are further strengthened by their use of the broad term *physical activity*, which can include activities as diverse as play, exercise, sport, dance and active living. This term is preferable to the narrower *exercise*, which is commonly perceived as involving hard work, strenuous activity and perhaps organised sport (and therefore seems unattractive or even intimidating to some young people). *Physical activity*, in contrast, is characterized by **flexibility** in that the activity can vary from day to day in terms of type, setting, intensity, duration and amount; it also affords various ways to meet the recommendations according to a child's stage of maturation. In addition, the recommendations promote a range of components of physical fitness, including muscular strength and aerobic fitness. Finally, they are reasonably straightforward and child friendly in comparison with some previous guidelines (some of which, for example, specified that activity intensity should fall within a specific range of percentage of maximum heart rate).

At the same time, the recommendations are marked by some limitations. For one thing, they are based on relatively limited research evidence and are subject to the fact that gaps exist in what we know about the association between physical activity and children's health (Cale & Harris, 2009). For example, it is difficult to precisely quantify minimal and optimal amounts of physical activity for young people. Therefore,

engaging in less activity than recommended does not necessarily mean that the activity will not be beneficial; to the contrary, any increase in physical activity may provide some health benefits for young people. As a result, simple messages such as 'some is better than none' and 'try to do a bit more' may lead to some of the same benefits and are likely to be more easily achievable by most.

The recommendations are also limited by the assumption that children will be able to make time, will wish to do so, or will find suitable opportunities to exercise frequently for as much as an hour a day. The commonly held view that children have ample time and energy for activity is debatable, especially for older children who must meet commitments at school, at home and possibly in part-time work positions. Therefore, even though physical activity can be accumulated throughout the day, the recommendations still require children to be sufficiently motivated and to either have or know how to make sufficient time for such activity.

Another limitation lies in the fact that the recommendations may not be well known among young people (HSCIC, 2008). In fact, it has been reported that only 10 percent of 12- to 15-year-olds in England were familiar with the recommendations for their age (Roth & Stamatakis, 2010). Moreover, the recommendations are not yet included in the formal curriculum of many schools.

Furthermore, confusion sometimes arises between recommendations for physical activity for health and government targets relating to how much time children should spend on PE and sport in schools. Examples of government targets include a previous long-term ambition in England to ensure that all children had two hours per week of curriculum physical education and the opportunity to access an additional two to three hours of sport beyond the curriculum. Similarly, the Northern Irish, Scottish and Welsh governments expected schools to work towards providing two hours per week of good-quality PE for each child, as well as opportunities to participate in at least two hours per week of extracurricular sport. Whilst government targets such as these are generally desirable, they usually set a standard significantly lower than the recommended hour per day of physical activity for health. At the same time, the two sets of recommendations support each other in that government targets for PE and sport in schools help ensure increased opportunities for children to achieve the recommended hour per day. We must also recognise, however, that children still need to be able to find ways of being active for at least two to three hours per week while away from school (e.g., in and around the home) whether with family or friends or on their own.

Given these various limitations, we propose viewing the recommendations as principles rather than strict rules, rigid prescriptions or unyielding standards. In other words, they should be seen as goals to progress towards rather than rigid standards dictating the same starting point and rate of progression for every child and forcing children to participate in a fixed regime of physical activity (Cale & Harris, 2009). In addition, they should be applied with both common sense and sensitivity, taking into account children's health and activity histories, physical fitness levels, functional capacities, personal circumstances, personalities, goals, preferences and dislikes. Finally, we advocate the view that all physical activity—including activity of light intensity (e.g., strolling, leisure walking)—provides health benefits when performed safely. As a result, there should be no hierarchy of activities, and pupils should be helped to learn to value all forms and types of physical activity.

A key area to focus on is how recommendations for physical activity for health are promoted, interpreted and accepted by teachers, health professionals, parents. Guidance for meeting physical activity recommendations for children include the following:

- Help pupils recognise barriers that restrict their physical activity (e.g., lack of time, money, facilities, transport) and find ways to overcome them.

- Help pupils appreciate the full range of physical activity opportunities available to them and identify effective ways to incorporate such activities into their daily lives (e.g., walking or cycling to school, shops or meetings with friends).

- Spread the word: disseminate and promote the recommendations and key messages to pupils, colleagues and other schools.

- Make best use of the opportunities and time provided through government targets to support the recommended one hour of physical activity per day.

- Enable the highest possible quality of PE and school sport experiences to motivate

pupils and encourage them to be active in their own time.

- Discuss with pupils the nature, scope and use of physical activity recommendations and share with them the limitations and cautions outlined in this chapter.

Finally, we recommend adopting an individualised, personalised and differentiated approach when giving pupils guidance about physical activity. Pupils should be encouraged to set attainable short-term goals and engage in types and amounts of physical activity that are appropriate for and appealing to them (Cale & Harris, 2009).

Fitness Testing Recommendations for Children

When exercise recommendations for young people were first formulated in the 1970s and 1980s, they tended to mirror recommendations made for adults in terms of specifying the volume of activity (i.e., frequency, intensity, time and type, as specified in the acronymic **FITT principle**) required to bring about changes in fitness test scores. For example, in 1988, the American College of Sports Medicine (ACSM) reported that children should undertake vigorous exercise every day for 20 to 30 minutes in order to experience fitness gains. The ACSM (1991, 1995) went on to provide practical advice for those involved in designing training programmes for children—for example, gradually increasing the quantity of exercise; ensuring adequate muscular strength and flexibility; using proper body mechanics, proper footwear and appropriate running surfaces; and taking precautions in high-temperature environments.

In the 1970s and 1980s, the considerable interest in fitness testing of children led to the development of fitness test batteries, such as, in 1976, the Youth Fitness Test provided by the American Alliance for Health, Physical Education and Recreation (AAHPER). Early test batteries such as this one faced some criticism because they predominantly tested motor fitness (including agility, balance, coordination and skill). Over time, they lost popularity and were replaced by different school-based programmes. For example, the Youth Fitness Test was replaced in 1988 by Physical Best, which was provided by the renamed American Alliance for Health, Physical Education, Recreation and Dance (AAHPERD).

Also in the 1980s, the Cooper Institute for Aerobics Research introduced Fitnessgram, which was intended to address concerns about fitness testing of children and resulted in more comprehensive fitness education programmes. Fitnessgram has since been successfully updated and further developed and is widely used as an education programme (Plowman et al., 2006; Morrow, Scott, Martin, & Jackson, 2010).

Over time, specific fitness recommendations for children came to be replaced by more holistic physical activity guidelines, such as the Children's Lifetime Physical Activity Model (Corbin, Pangrazi, & Welk, 1994). This model proposed, as a minimum, that children should engage in daily moderate physical activity for 30 minutes or more spread across three or more sessions per day through childhood games and lifestyle activities (e.g., walking to school). Four years later, in England, the Health Education Authority established recommendations for young people which have since been replaced by UK-wide physical activity guidelines for children and young people aged 5 to 18 years (Department of Health; Department of Health, Social Sciences and Public Safety; Scottish Government; Welsh Government; 2011). These newer guidelines state the following:

1. All children and young people should engage in moderate to vigorous intensity physical activity for at least 60 minutes and up to several hours every day.

2. Vigorous intensity activities, including those that strengthen muscle and bone, should be incorporated at least three days a week.

3. All children and young people should minimise the amount of time spent being sedentary (sitting) for extended periods.

The 2011 UK-wide physical activity guidelines differed from the previous guidelines for this age in the following ways:

- Inclusion of vigorous physical activity in recognition of the additional benefits it can provide
- Emphasis of 60 minutes per day as a minimum with the addition of the statement 'and up to several hours every day'
- Increased frequency of activities to strengthen muscle and bone (from two days to at least three days per week)

- Omission of a guideline relating to flexibility
- Addition of a guideline relating to minimizing sedentary behaviour

These guidelines sit alongside the similar WHO recommendations outlined earlier in this chapter. Both recommend at least one hour of moderate to vigorous physical activity per day for 5- to 17-year-olds and encourage vigorous activities that strengthen muscle and bone at least three times per week. The two sets of recommendations differ only in that the WHO guidelines explicitly state that physical activity of amounts greater than 60 minutes per day will provide additional health benefits, whereas the UK guidelines state that all children and young people should minimise time spent being sedentary (sitting) for extended periods. Given their similarities, both sets of recommendations are advocated for use in schools. As discussed earlier, the recommendations are characterized by both strengths and limitations, and we advise taking care to implement them sensitively and wisely.

A quiz titled Children's Health, Activity and Fitness Recommendations is available for printing or completing electronically in the web resource. This quiz has been created for use with children in upper primary or lower secondary school. It includes a series of questions based on health recommendations associated with nutrition and physical activity. The questions address points

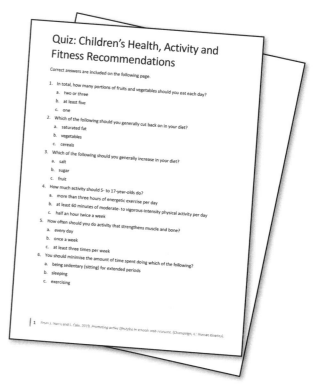

such as how much of one's diet should consist of fruits and vegetables each day and how much activity should be done by children aged 5 to 17 years; answers are included. The quiz can be used to gauge children's knowledge and understanding of common health guidelines before teaching them about healthy eating and active living.

Common Misconceptions About Children's Health, Activity and Fitness

Studies over a number of decades and from across the world have shown that children hold misconceptions and misunderstandings about health, activity and fitness (Brusseau, Kulinna, & Cothran, 2011; Burrows & Wright, 2004; Burrows, Wright, & Jungersen-Smith, 2002; Dixey, Sahota, Atwal, & Turner, 2001; Harris, 1993, 1994; Harris, Cale, Duncombe, & Musson, 2016; Keating et al., 2009; Merkle & Treagust, 1993; O'Shea & Beausoleil, 2012; Placek et al., 2001; Powell & Fitzpatrick, 2015; Stewart & Mitchell, 2003). For example, children tend to consider health almost exclusively in a physical or corporeal sense (predominantly in terms of body shape and size) and view food and exercise as the main moderators of health. They also tend to describe health from a negative perspective, stating what they should avoid doing in order to stay healthy (e.g., eating sugary or fatty foods, being sedentary for long periods) rather than what they should do. These findings suggest that children tend to have a somewhat narrow and negative perspective on what it means to be healthy.

These studies also provide evidence of worrying gaps, and some confusion, in young people's knowledge and understanding of health, fitness and physical activity. For example, many young people

- think that fitness is about being thin and looking good,
- think that exercise must be hard in order to be good,
- fail to make informed links between exercise or energy expenditure and being overweight or obese and

- have only a superficial understanding of the relationship between health and exercise.

It has been suggested that young people's inadequate or inaccurate understandings of health, fitness and physical activity may result from how these subjects are taught in schools and addressed in popular culture (Burrows & Wright, 2004; Burrows et al., 2002; Lee & Macdonald, 2009, 2010). This may be true, for instance, of approaches steeped in 'healthism' discourse, which is based on the notion that health can be achieved 'unproblematically through individual effort and discipline, directed mainly at regulating the size and shape of the body' (Crawford, cited in Kirk and Colquhoun, 1989, p. 419). Such approaches may lead young people to develop reductive, limited and limiting conceptualisations of health, fitness and physical activity (Burrows, 2008; Burrows & Wright, 2004; Burrows et al., 2002; Burrows, Wright, & McCormack, 2009; Harris et al., 2016; Lee & Macdonald, 2009, 2010). Moreover, young people's engagement with healthism discourses may be facilitated by well-meaning but inadequately prepared teachers who themselves hold narrow, reductive views of health, fitness and physical activity (Harris et al., 2016; Lee & Macdonald, 2009, 2010). Such cases may result in schools falling well short of their potential to promote healthy, active lifestyles.

This danger implies an urgent need to increase the breadth, depth and relevance of young people's learning about health in schools. Specifically, a coordinated whole-school approach to teaching health would help young people connect learning across a range of subjects. In addition, we can adopt teaching approaches that help pupils relate their learning to themselves and their everyday lives. In PE, in particular, learning should challenge the narrow focus, misunderstandings and misconceptions that many young people hold concerning health, fitness and physical activity. Meeting this goal is likely to require us to develop alternative approaches, both in initial teacher education and in professional development related to PE-for-health pedagogies. Approaches that address pupils' misunderstandings and misconceptions are presented in parts 2 and 3 of this book. You can also visit the web resource for a printable handout titled Debunking Myths and Misconceptions About Children's Health, Activity and Fitness.

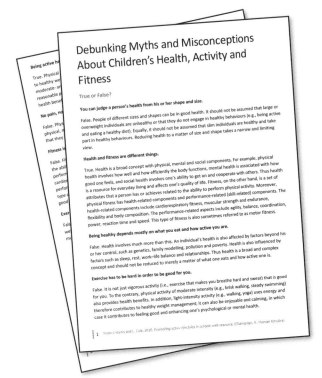

Debunking Myths and Misconceptions About Children's Health, Activity and Fitness

True or False?

You can judge a person's health from his or her shape and size.

False. People of different sizes and shapes can be in good health. It should not be assumed that large or overweight individuals are unhealthy or that they do not engage in healthy behaviours (e.g., being active and eating a healthy diet). Equally, it should not be assumed that slim individuals are healthy and take part in healthy behaviours. Reducing health to a matter of size and shape takes a narrow and limiting view.

Health and fitness are different things.

True. Health is a broad concept with physical, mental and social components. For example, physical health involves how well and how efficiently the body functions, mental health is associated with how good one feels, and social health involves one's ability to get on and cooperate with others. Thus health is a resource for everyday living and affects one's quality of life. Fitness, on the other hand, is a set of attributes that a person has or achieves related to the ability to perform physical activity. Moreover, physical fitness has health-related components and performance-related (skill-related) components. The health-related components include cardiorespiratory fitness, muscular strength and endurance, flexibility and body composition. The performance-related aspects include agility, balance, coordination, power, reaction time and speed. This type of fitness is also sometimes referred to as motor fitness.

Being healthy depends mostly on what you eat and how active you are.

False. Health involves much more than this. An individual's health is also affected by factors beyond his or her control, such as genetics, family modelling, pollution and poverty. Health is also influenced by factors such as sleep, rest, work–life balance and relationships. Thus health is a broad and complex concept and should not be reduced to merely a matter of what one eats and how active one is.

Exercise has to be hard in order to be good for you.

False. It is not just vigorous activity (i.e., exercise that makes you breathe hard and sweat) that is good for you. To the contrary, physical activity of moderate intensity (e.g., brisk walking, steady swimming) also provides health benefits. In addition, light-intensity activity (e.g., walking, yoga) uses energy and therefore contributes to healthy weight management; it can also be enjoyable and calming, in which case it contributes to feeling good and enhancing one's psychological or mental health.

1   From J. Harris and L. Cale, 2018, *Promoting active lifestyles in schools web resource.* (Champaign, IL: Human Kinetics).

Summary

The rationale for promoting physical activity among children has been strengthened in recent decades, both by the growing evidence of the benefits of physical activity in childhood and by the increased prevalence of inactivity-related health conditions among children. Schools provide important avenues through which to promote healthy lifestyles, as they reach virtually all children and provide structured, progressive programmes taught by professionals. In particular, school PE can play a key role in promoting active ways of life. To help promote active lifestyles, we encourage you to make effective use of well-established recommendations for activity by children (at least one hour per day) and to be mindful of the limitations of a 'one size fits all' or testing-dominated approach in the school setting. We also advise you to incorporate approaches that address gaps, misunderstandings and misconceptions in children's knowledge and understanding of health, fitness and physical activity.

Whole-School Approaches to Promoting Healthy Lifestyles

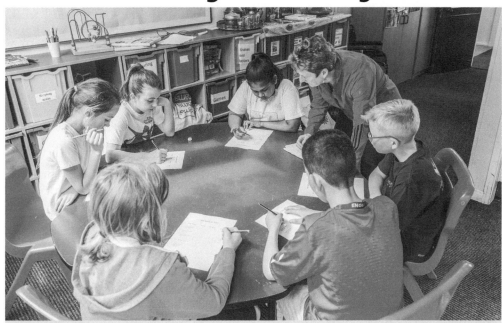

Chapter Objectives

After reading this chapter, you will be able to

- ▶ describe whole-school approaches (e.g., healthy-school programmes) to enhancing health behaviours;
- ▶ appreciate the multidimensional nature of health in its physical, psychological and social aspects, which involve individuals, groups, communities and the environment;
- ▶ recognise various approaches to health education that draw from selected health behaviour theories and models;
- ▶ identify active schools that explicitly commit to maximising opportunities for all adults and children in school to be active;
- ▶ make use of active pedagogies in lessons and activity breaks during the school day to increase pupils' activity levels in the school setting; and
- ▶ understand that promoting activity involves collaboration among all who exercise significant influence on pupils.

Healthy schools aim to achieve healthy lifestyles for the entire school population—pupils; teaching, support and administrative staff; governors; and parents—by developing a supportive environment conducive to the promotion of health. A healthy school depends on three key elements: curriculum, environment (or 'hidden' curriculum) and community. In addition, a healthy school is committed to promoting good health through its curricular, extracurricular and organisational practices.

Whole-school approaches to encouraging and enhancing health behaviours have emerged as a global priority (Stewart-Brown, 2006). As a result, whole-school initiatives have been designed and implemented in many countries to help create schools that

- identify health as a central feature of the school agenda;
- foster positive attitudes towards health among staff and pupils;
- reinforce and reward health knowledge and understanding and healthy behaviour;
- acknowledge that behaviour is influenced by a range of factors that go beyond simply holding individuals responsible for their health and activity; and
- share responsibility for promoting healthy lifestyles and encourage working in partnership to enhance health.

Creating a Healthy School

Back in the late 1990s, the National Healthy Schools Programme was launched by the government in England to raise awareness of school opportunities to improve the health of children, teachers, families and the local community. The initial version of the programme included national quality standards for healthy schools based on a number of health themes, one of which was physical activity. In order to achieve in this area, schools had to demonstrate that they

- took a whole-school approach to promoting physical activity;
- offered all pupils, regardless of age or ability, at least two hours of physical activity per week within and two hours outside the curriculum;

- were aware of a range of relevant initiatives and networks and took advantage of appropriate opportunities to promote and develop physical activity; and
- encouraged staff, parents and other adults to become more involved in promoting physical activity and helped them develop their skills, abilities and understanding through appropriate training.

(Department for Education and Employment, 1999)

As part of this programme, a toolkit was designed to help schools 'plan, do and review' health and well-being improvements for their pupils and identify and select effective activities and interventions (Department of Health, 2005). The 'plan' phase included selecting health and well-being priorities based on data about pupils' needs, defining outcomes and identifying possible activities and interventions to achieve those outcomes. The 'do' phase involved selecting and implementing activities and interventions to help achieve the desired outcomes, monitoring progress towards the outcomes and making any necessary adjustments to milestones and outcomes. The 'review' phase required schools to evaluate achievement of outcomes, share and celebrate improvements in pupils' health and well-being and review the provision of programming to promote health and well-being.

Another national approach to developing healthy schools has been mounted in Wales through the Welsh Network of Healthy School Schemes. This effort, launched in 1999, uses National Quality Award indicators relating to seven key health topics: food and fitness, emotional health and well-being, personal development and relationships, substance use and misuse, environment, safety and hygiene. The indicators for these health topics are expressed in the following aspects of school life (Welsh Assembly Government, 2009).

- Leadership and communication: policy developed by a working group that includes pupils; evidence of complementary roles of policy and curriculum; appropriate training for teachers; school engagement with and support of community initiatives
- Curriculum: schemes of work that identify physical activity, oral health and nutrition (including links between food and fitness and mental and emotional health and well-

being) and reflect policy; school commitment to providing two hours of high-quality PE per week for every pupil; provisions of consistent messages (and avoidance of mixed messages) in relation to diet, oral health and physical activity

- Ethos and environment: evidence of food and fitness initiatives that actively involve pupils; encouragement of all staff to demonstrate behaviours consistent with policy on food and fitness; environment that encourages physical activity
- Family and community involvement: well-informed parents and governors who understand the importance of policy on good nutrition and physical activity, for both pupils and themselves; links with local community organisations, sport clubs and businesses to support the food and fitness agenda; use of expertise from parents and community members to support curricular or, if appropriate, noncurricular activities

Similarly, in 2004, Scotland launched a national framework for health-promoting schools under the banner of Being Well—Doing Well. This approach identifies key characteristics of health-promoting schools in relation to the following areas: leadership and management; ethos; partnership working; curriculum, learning and teaching; personal, social, health and economic education programmes; and environment, resources and facilities (Scottish Health Promoting Schools Unit, 2004). In 2008, the Schools (Health Promotion and Nutrition) (Scotland) Act published further guidance for schools, which described health-promoting schools as those that

- ensure entitlement to and participation in physically healthy activities for all, particularly those who are less active;
- embed physical activity within the school development plan;
- build PE into a whole-school approach to promoting health and physical activity

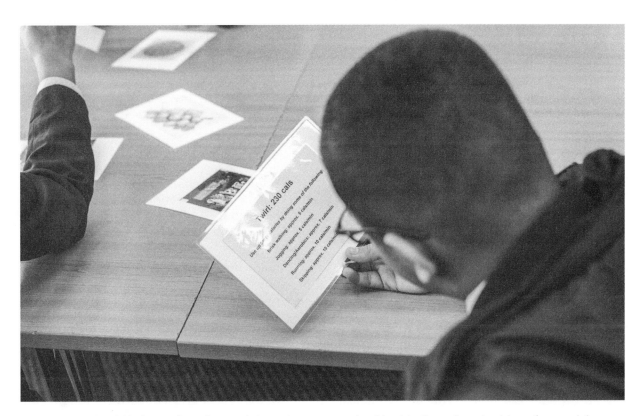

Programmes should help pupils understand the various ways to lead healthy lives; they should not focus solely on exercise and sport.

across the curriculum, most notably in PE, physical activity and sport but also, for example, in the sciences (e.g., beneficial effects of regular exercise, need for good personal hygiene and dental hygiene) and in mathematics (e.g., BMI, comparing energy intake and energy expenditure);

- maximise opportunities for pupils to be active in the classroom throughout the school day in order to improve concentration and focus for learning;

- help pupils understand that physical activity can be incorporated into all aspects of school life, and life beyond school, through such activities as walking to and from school or work, attending a dance class, playing outside with friends, rambling and cycling;

- provide opportunities and space for physical activity, play, eating, socialising and privacy;

- ensure that school grounds are clean, safe and maintained to a high standard in order to encourage pupils to be physically active;

- promote active travel, such as walking and cycling to school, and provide cycle racks, secure lockers and appropriate areas for changing and showering; and

- provide physical activity opportunities through wider school and community activities to allow young people to be physically active in less formal settings and to give them more choice and influence regarding the types of activities in which they participate (Scottish Government, 2008).

Northern Ireland has a similar programme, known as Health Action Schools, which was set up in 2003 by Action Cancer. This programme is designed to improve knowledge of health and encourage pupils to take ownership of their lifestyle choices. It also provides gold, silver and bronze Health Action awards to schools. The programme for nursery schools introduces pupils to 'golden rules' for being healthy in relation to eating, exercise, smoking and sun safety. The primary-school programme focuses on the dangers of smoking and of drinking alcohol; the importance of eating a healthy, balanced diet; the effects of being physically active; and ways to stay safe in the sun. The programme for secondary school includes workshop-based sessions that cover healthy eating, exercise, cancer awareness, smoking and alcohol.

Health Education Models and Approaches

Health education provides planned opportunities for participants to develop knowledge and life skills conducive to individual and community health. It views health as a multidimensional phenomenon including mental, physical, spiritual and emotional aspects and concerning individuals, groups, communities and the environment. Health education can be implemented through a variety of approaches drawing from a range of health behaviour theories and models. Here are selected approaches considered relevant to the school setting.

- Rational model: Also known as the 'knowledge, attitudes, practices' model, this approach is based on the premise that increasing a person's knowledge will lead to changes in attitude and behaviour. It is now generally considered to be a somewhat simplistic model of behaviour change.

- Health belief model: This more complex approach centres on the premise that health-related decision making and behaviour are based on a range of factors, including perceived susceptibility to an identified threat, severity of the threat, benefits and barriers, cues to action and self-efficacy.

- Transtheoretical model of change: This model views behaviour change in terms of progression through five stages of readiness to change: precontemplation (not thinking about change), contemplation (starting to think about change), preparation (ready to take action), action (making changes in behaviour) and maintenance (sustaining behaviour change).

- Theory of planned behaviour: This approach holds that intent is influenced not only by one's attitude towards behaviour but also by one's perception of social norms (i.e., the strength of others' opinions about the behaviour and one's own motivation to comply with the opinions of significant others) and one's degree of perceived behavioural control.

- Activated health education model: This three-phase model holds particular relevance for schools. The first phase, which is experiential, actively engages individuals in assessing their health. The second phase, which involves awareness, presents information and creates awareness of the target behaviour. The third phase, which focuses on responsibility, helps individuals identify personal responsibility, clarify personal health values and develop a customised plan for behaviour change.

Based on World Health Organization 2012.

These approaches go some way towards conveying the challenge of health behaviour change, which involves a complex interplay of knowledge, understanding and attitudes and is influenced by social norms. Awareness of these approaches can help you make appropriate decisions about how to deliver health-related topics. These decisions can facilitate curriculum-focused outcomes that go well beyond increased knowledge and understanding and include the development of particular skills and attributes, as well as enhanced attitudes towards adopting healthy lifestyles.

Active Schools Models and Approaches

The same three elements that have traditionally formed the basis of a healthy schools model—curriculum, environment and community—are also important in an active schools model. An active school is expected to commit explicitly to physical activity and to maximise opportunities for activity among all adults and children associated with the school (Cale, 1997; Fox, 1996; McMullen, Ni Chroinin, Tammelin, Pogorzelska, & Van der Mars, 2015). The first steps recommended in seeking to become an active school are to develop an active-school policy and set up an active-school committee. Here is an example of an active-school policy.

Curriculum

- Allocate at least two hours per week of curriculum time for PE for all pupils.
- Provide a broad, balanced, relevant and high-quality PE programme that complies with statutory requirements and is accessible to and meets the needs and interests of all pupils.
- Fully implement health-related PE requirements through a programme of study that is effectively structured, planned, delivered and evaluated.
- Promote physical activity throughout the curriculum.
- Monitor pupils' levels of involvement in sport and activity (both in and out of school).
- Reduce the proportion of nonparticipating pupils in PE.
- Provide an extracurricular programme that includes a broad range of purposeful and enjoyable physical activities (e.g., competitive and noncompetitive, team and individual).
- Increase the proportion of pupils who regularly participate in extracurricular activities.
- Increase the proportion of staff who regularly contribute to the extracurricular programme.
- Organise events (in both curricular and extracurricular time) that promote physical activity (e.g., sport days, activity weeks, taster sessions).
- Identify both quantitative and qualitative targets related to health in PE development plans.

Environment (Hidden Curriculum)

- Provide areas for play that are safe, adequate and stimulating (both indoors and outdoors).
- Ensure that sport and activity facilities are adequate and well maintained.
- Make sport facilities and equipment available for recreational use at lunch and break times.
- Create inclusive, eye-catching displays and noticeboards about PE, sport and physical activity around the PE department and school.

Community

- Raise awareness among and enlist support from staff, parents, governors and community members for the physical activity messages promoted in school.
- Provide all pupils with accurate, up-to-date information about the activity opportunities available in the local community.
- Provide opportunities for pupils, staff, governors and parents to be active.

- Develop alliances and partnerships with local providers (e.g., sport clubs, leisure centres) to increase opportunities for activity.
- Formulate an active-school committee (with pupil, staff, governor and parent representatives) to develop, implement and evaluate the effectiveness of the active-school policy.

Adapted, by permission, from L. Cale and J. Harris, 2009, *Getting the buggers fit* (London: Continuum), 160-161. Used by permission of Bloomsbury Publishing Plc.

These models help ensure that activity promotion is given high status and placed firmly on the school agenda. They can also help you develop a clear vision (in terms of goals and objectives to increase activity), identify the means for realising that vision, and coordinate and evaluate physical activity strategies and initiatives in the school. Instead of creating separate policies, schools can incorporate physical activity objectives and elements of an active-school policy into existing, related policies. As every school is different—for example, in its location, composition and resources—the content of any policy should focus primarily on the needs of the school's staff and pupils. Moreover, the goals and strategies emanating from the policy should be realistic and feasible.

One flexible approach to promoting physical activity is to adopt key principles that can be applied in a range of ways in different schools. The following list presents 10 PAL (promoting active lifestyles) principles, some or all of which schools may be able to apply, depending on their particular circumstances (for more about PAL, see chapter 3).

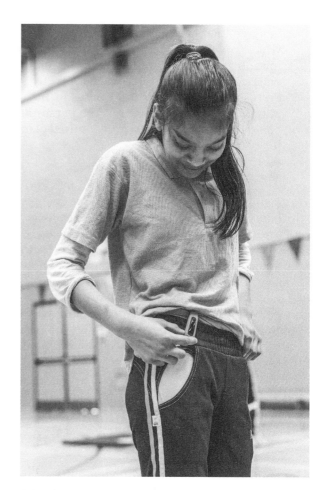

Schools can encourage pupils to become more active by integrating the use of activity trackers which provide a clear visual account of activity during the day.

1. Include guidelines for physical activity for health among children in both physical education and PSHE education (alongside other health guidelines).

2. Discuss the promotion of active lifestyles, including marketing the 'one hour a day' physical activity guideline, with all staff, governors, pupils and parents.

3. Make the goal of increasing physical activity levels an agenda item for school councils and encourage pupil representatives to propose ideas for achieving it.

4. Increase activity levels in non-PE lessons by having pupils move more within the learning environment (e.g., in the classroom or outdoors).

5. Promote active travel to school (e.g., cycling, walking, scooting) and ensure safe storage of cycles and scooters.

6. Ensure that physical activity facilities (including changing areas) are clean, safe and well managed.

7. Review the school's extracurricular physical activity programme and consider how accessible and appealing it is for *all* pupils.

8. Encourage teachers from all subjects to contribute to the school's extracurricular programme; when they do, reward them.

9. Visibly raise the profile of physical activity in school (e.g., via noticeboards, newsletters, intranet or website, assemblies, in-school screens and videos).

10. Develop good community links (e.g., with feeder or partner schools, local leisure centres and sport clubs) to increase the quality and quantity of physical activity opportunities for pupils.

Increasing Activity Levels in All Lessons

To build on physical activity provided in the PE curriculum and the extracurricular programme, schools should consider increasing physical activity across all areas of the curriculum (e.g., in English, maths and science lessons). This approach is consistent with the active schools philosophy, which aims to maximise opportunities for all adults and children in the school to be active. With this end in mind, in recent years, standing desks have been trialled in schools to help address sedentary behaviour, and studies in England and Australia have found that the use of standing desks in primary schools resulted in more in-class activity (Clemes et al., 2015). Some schools have also purchased activity trackers (e.g., pedometers) to encourage increased physical activity during the school day. Pedometers have been used in programmes such as Schools on the Move (Youth Sport Trust, Department for Education and Skills and Department of Health), which have found them effective in increasing physical activity among the school population (Lubans, Morgan, & Tudor-Locke, 2009; Stathi, Nordin, & Riddoch, 2006).

Active Cross-Curricular Links

Cross-curricular links with an activity focus can help increase the amount of time for which pupils are physically active during the school day; they can also provide a different, stimulating environment for effective learning (British Heart Foundation, 1999b). In addition, such links can help pupils connect health-related learning in various subjects—for example, the effects of exercise on the body, which is often taught in both physical education and science lessons. These connections can make the learning experience more coherent for pupils and improve the effectiveness of their learning. Ideas for increasing physical activity across the curriculum can be generated through liaison among subject leaders at the school. Here are some examples.

- Mapping activities in humanities lessons (e.g., locating markers or geocaches in the school grounds or local area)
- Science investigations, such as changes to pulse rate and breathing intensity during various activities (e.g., walking, jogging, skipping, walking up stairs)
- Nature walks in science lessons
- Measurement activities in mathematics lessons (e.g., monitoring distances covered when walking, jogging, running or jumping)
- Activities to develop literacy and numeracy in PE lessons

Active Pedagogies

Schools can also encourage the adoption of teaching approaches that increase pupils' activity levels during lessons. Such approaches, known as **active pedagogies**, use tasks that involve children in moving within the learning environment. One method to help pupils become more active is simply to have them answer a question (e.g., How active should people of your age be?) by moving to the most appropriate response among a range of options (only one of which is correct) placed on large cards located in various parts of the learning area. You can tailor the questions, answers and follow-up discussions differently for different age groups. For example, in working with pupils aged 7 through 11 years, you might use the following question:

How often should you be active?

For this question, the answers written on the cards could be as follows: once a week, every day, twice a week, every other day, on school days only. The simplicity of the question and the broad time frames given in the answers match the level of complexity and understanding of younger pupils. The follow-up for pupils in this age range might be to inform them that they should be active every day for an hour or more and that this time can be made up of shorter periods of time (e.g., four 15-minute blocks or six 10-minute blocks). An associated numeracy challenge could be provided by asking the children to calculate different ways in which the one hour could be accumulated.

This challenge should include energetic activities, including some that strengthen bones and muscles.

When working with pupils aged 11 through 14 years, the following question and answers might be used to appeal to their ability to conceptualise at higher levels:

> How much activity should people of your age do?

Answer-station cards for this question could include the following: 10 minutes of energetic activity every day, one hour of energetic activity each day, 30 minutes of activity every day, two hours of activity per week, 5 minutes of very energetic activity daily. In the follow-up discussion, young people should be made aware that one hour of energetic physical activity is the minimum recommendation for good health and that it should include some activities that strengthen muscles and bones. You could also point out to them that the responses indicating 5, 10 and 30 minutes of activity, respectively, could be part of the 'one hour a day' made up of multiple accumulated time blocks. You could also replace the term 'energetic' in the 'one hour a day' response with 'moderate- to vigorous-intensity' if the young people have been taught these concepts. In the United Kingdom, many young people experience two hours of PE per week, and they should understand that this time contributes to the recommended amount of physical activity per week but falls well short of it (by five hours).

Another method of increasing physical activity levels during lessons is to ask pupils to respond to a series of statements (e.g., PE is good fun; I hate fitness testing) by moving to the most appropriate response among a set of options spaced around the learning environment. The available responses might include *agree*, *not sure* and *disagree* for pupils aged 7 through 11 years and *strongly agree*, *agree*, *not sure* (or *don't know* or *neutral*), *disagree* and *strongly disagree* for pupils aged 11 through 14 years. Here are some examples of statements and related discussions.

Response Statements for Pupils Aged 7 to 11

Children's responses to the following statements can be used to trigger discussions about what they like (and dislike) about PE and about the range of active choices available during breaks and lunchtimes.

- PE is good fun.
- I get bored during break times.
- I enjoy going to after-school activity and sport clubs.
- I look forward to my PE lessons.
- There is not much to do at lunchtimes.

Response Statements for Pupils Aged 11 to 14

Young people's responses to the following statements can be used to trigger discussions about what they like (and dislike) about fitness testing and should also reveal their understanding of the relationships between fitness, activity and health. Young people should be informed that being active provides health benefits and can lead to improved fitness and that they should aim to be active for at least one hour per day. To see if they are meeting this recommendation, you might also encourage them to keep an activity diary for a period of time.

- Fitness testing is enjoyable.
- Fitness testing is a good way to find out how active you are.
- We should be fitness-tested every term of every year.
- Fitness testing is good for you.
- I hate fitness testing.

Another way to use active pedagogies in the classroom is to ask pupils to demonstrate their understanding of a topic or concept by moving to various locations in the learning area. For example, pupils might be asked to collect items from around the room that are environmentally friendly. Here are some examples for two different age groups:

Suggested Tasks for Pupils Aged 7 to 11

- Move to the equipment you need to use next.
- Touch five items in the room that are made of plastic (or wood or metal).
- Take your partner to the picture or photograph that you like best and tell him or her why you like it so much.
- Move around the area and choose a tree (or shrub or flower) that you would like to sketch. Then collect the equipment needed for sketching and set yourself up to start.

- In a group of three, act out how the sun, earth and moon move in relation to each other.

Suggested Tasks for Pupils Aged 11 to 14

- Move around the room and rate the various items or products (according to indicated criteria). Then take your group to the items or products that you have rated the highest (first and second) and explain why you rated them so highly.
- Have each person in your group select one item in the area to use in a group design. Show your selected items to the group and explain why you chose them. As a group, discuss whether—and if so, how—each item could be used in the group design.
- As part of your warm-up, use five ways of travelling on your feet while progressing gradually from first 'gear' to fifth.
- Choose one photograph from those on display around the room. Think of a story that could be associated with this photograph. Take your partner to see your selected photograph and tell her or him your story.
- Collect matching items from around the room, as well as one that does not match. Ask your group to work out and explain which items match and why—and which item is the odd one out.

Activity Breaks

Another way to increase pupils' physical activity participation is to incorporate activity breaks within the school day (British Heart Foundation, 1999a). Teachers who have used this approach have reported positive responses from pupils, including increased concentration and improved behaviour (Donnelly, 2011). To help maximise learning time, these breaks can be associated with key concepts or health messages. Here are a few possibilities.

- Incorporating an active start to, or component within, each lesson, as seen in the examples provided in the previous section on active pedagogies
- Informing pupils about the next topic or task during a walk outside
- Asking pupils to perform actions in the classroom (with or without music) that are associated with a series of health messages such as 'an hour a day keeps the doctor at bay'. An example for this particular message could include a sequence of actions designed to represent 'an hour', 'a day', 'doctor' and 'keep...at bay'.

Here are some examples of heart-health messages for 7- through 11-year-olds:

- Being active is good for your heart.
- Activity strengthens your muscles and bones.
- Being active should be a daily habit, like brushing your teeth.
- Move more; sit less.
- Active children are happy children.

And here are some examples of heart-health messages for 11- through 14-year-olds:

- An hour a day keeps the doctor at bay.
- Some activity is better than none.
- Get into a habit of activity—it all adds up.
- Excellence in PE is maintaining an active lifestyle.
- Friends who are active together stick together.

- Asking pupils to lead exercises for their peers
- Asking pupils to sing and move to action songs, such as 'Head, Shoulders, Knees and Toes' (and to progress to creating their own action songs)
- Asking pupils to play simple action games, such as Simon Says (and to progress to creating their own action games)
- Asking pupils to design actions for use with popular music and teach them to peers or younger pupils

A number of organisations have provided activity ideas for the classroom, hall or playground. Examples include Take 10—Fit to Succeed and Take 10—Every Move Counts (Devon Local Authority), Activators Cards (Norfolk County Council), Class Moves (Welsh Assembly Government and NHS Health Scotland) and 10 Minute Shake Up resources (Public Health England, 2017). Though some of these ideas have yet to be formally evaluated, findings regarding those that have been studied suggest that they can help increase the physical activity levels of all pupils in the school setting (Lowden, Powney, Davidson, & James, 2001).

Activity breaks should be seen not as a replacement for curriculum physical education but as a complement to it. School PE lessons provide the means by which pupils learn to become physically competent in a broad range of physical activities and develop valuable transferable skills such as cooperation, collaboration, teamwork, perseverance and resilience. This learning must not be replaced with activity breaks.

Working With Parents to Promote Active Lifestyles

A holistic approach to promoting active lifestyles involves collaboration among all those who exert significant influence on pupils, including parents and other family members (e.g., siblings, grandparents). Research indicates that children and young people are more likely to be active if their parents and other family members are active,

HEALTHIER TOGETHER

An inner-city secondary school and its eight feeder primary schools decided to make a concerted effort to work with parents to promote healthy lifestyles in the local community. The initiative, known as Healthier Together, was proposed by a member of the senior school management team and discussed with governors to ensure high-level approval from the outset. In collaboration with parent–teacher committees, a programme flier was developed to outline the schools' ambition of promoting healthy behaviours among pupils and their families and to describe the plan for achieving this goal. The flier also included information about the benefits of healthy lifestyles and the possible consequences of unhealthy ways of life. It was shared with all staff and parents in the respective schools.

> **Discussion point:** How important do you think it is to involve parents in the development of such an initiative, and why?

In addition, organisers distributed a calendar of Healthier Together events scheduled for the academic year. These events included activity and healthy-eating events involving pupils and their families—for example, a Jolly January Jog, a Summer Sunset Stroll and a Healthy Bake-Off.

> **Discussion point:** What are some other ideas for family-oriented events to promote and support healthy living?

The initiative also included a call-out (via website, e-mail and text) for parents to support extracurricular school activities and sports by assisting with supervision, equipment, refreshments and kit. Parents were also asked if they had any expertise or other qualifications in various activities and sports or would be willing to obtain a suitable qualification (with partial funding) in order to contribute to extracurricular sessions.

> **Discussion points:** What are your views on involving parents in delivering or supporting extracurricular sessions? What quality-assurance issues would schools need to consider in order to ensure the safety and well-being of their pupils?

The schools ran the initiative for a full school year and then evaluated its success, both in terms of increasing awareness and uptake of healthy behaviours among pupils, parents and in terms of increasing involvement of parents in extracurricular programmes. The evaluation took the form of discussions among staff in the participating schools and among the members of parent–teacher committees. In general, the initiative was considered to be successful both in improving awareness of healthy lifestyles among pupils and in increasing involvement of parents in supporting extracurricular programmes. From the nine schools, 11 parents were partially funded to obtain an exercise or coaching qualification, and 10 went on to deliver activity sessions in a number of the schools. This participation meant that the schools' extracurricular programmes could be extended to involve more pupils.

> **Discussion point:** What are your thoughts about how the initiative was evaluated?

although this result is certainly not guaranteed (Gustafson & Rhodes, 2006; Jago, Fox, Page, Brockman, & Thompson, 2010). Schools may consider liaising with parents in any of the following ways:

- Informing them about the school's policy to promote active lifestyles and how it plans to do so with their cooperation
- Educating them about the benefits of an active lifestyle and the possible consequences of a sedentary way of life (as in the Information Sheet for Parents available in the web resource for this chapter)
- Explaining guidelines for physical activity for health and how parents can help their children meet those guidelines (possibly using support resources such as the Get Kids on the Go booklet described in chapter 3)
- Encouraging an active way of life, including activities for the whole family (e.g., walking, swimming, cycling)
- Organising fun activity events that involve pupils and their families (e.g., Jolly Jog, Winter Waddle, Spring Steps, Summer Stroll)
- Encouraging support for school activities and sport events (e.g., helping with transport, equipment, refreshments and kit)
- Asking if they have qualifications or expertise related to activities or sports and would like to contribute to the school's extracurricular physical activity programme
- Asking if they would be willing to attain a suitable qualification (with partial funding) in order to make a regular commitment to delivering extracurricular physical activity sessions

Through effective communication with parents—via newsletters, websites, e-mail, texts and meetings—you can tap into a potentially vast source of goodwill and expertise. Doing so may allow you to increase the physical activity opportunities available to all pupils in the school setting.

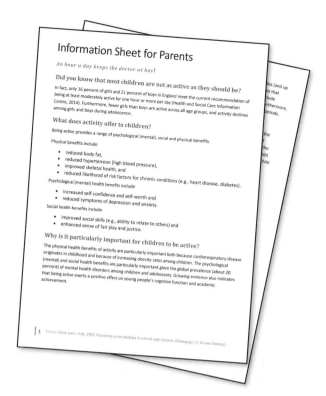

Summary

The various approaches to health education in schools reflect the multidimensional nature of health and convey the complexity and challenge involved in changing health behaviours. We encourage whole-school approaches, which help achieve healthy lifestyles for the entire school population through the curriculum, the environment and the community. Similarly, an active school maximises opportunities for all adults and children associated with the school to be active. To do so, it builds on physical activity in the PE curriculum and extracurricular programme by increasing physical activity across the curriculum. This expansion can be achieved by incorporating activity breaks within the school day that are associated with key health messages and encouraging the adoption of active teaching approaches or pedagogies. Schools should also pursue multiple ways to involve parents in promoting active lifestyles because, in order to be truly effective, our efforts should involve collaboration among all who exert a significant influence on children.

Physical Education's Contribution to Promoting Healthy Lifestyles

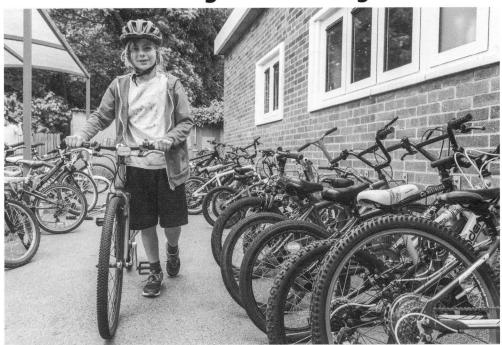

Chapter Objectives

After reading this chapter, you will be able to

▶ explain the rationale for increasing promotion of active lifestyles in physical education curricula;

▶ identify the knowledge, understanding, skills and attitudes associated with active lifestyles that can be taught in curriculum PE;

▶ identify ways to assess health-related learning;

▶ describe effective approaches to promoting active lifestyles in PE that result in affective, behavioural and cognitive (ABC) learning outcomes;

▶ recognise gaps between health-related rhetoric and reality that have led to calls for critical pedagogies, known collectively as 'PE for health', that are sociocultural and evidence-based; and

▶ use the support available for health-related learning in the form of programmes, resources and professional development.

This chapter explains the increasing promotion of active lifestyles in PE curricula and details the health-related learning that can be incorporated into school PE. You will be guided to select from a range of effective approaches to promoting active lifestyles in PE that avoid gaps between health-related rhetoric and reality. You will also be pointed towards relevant sources of support for this area of work.

Promoting Active Lifestyles in Curriculum Physical Education

The promotion of active lifestyles has been a key aim of PE curricula in the United Kingdom and around the world for many decades. For example, one main aim of the national curriculum for England is to ensure that all pupils lead healthy, active lives. In order to achieve this goal, 11- to 14-year-old pupils should develop the confidence and interest to get involved in exercise, sports and activities outside of school and in later life; they should also understand and pursue the long-term benefits of physical activity. Similarly, 14- to 16-year-olds should get involved in a range of activities that develop personal fitness and promote active, healthy lifestyles (Department for Education, 2013). Here are some examples of promoting active lifestyles in the PE curricula of other UK countries:

- The national curriculum for physical education in Northern Ireland states that PE should help young people develop positive attitudes towards participation in physical activities in their pursuit of healthy lifestyles. It also states that PE should help individuals develop awareness of the positive impact of physical activity on health and well-being (Council for the Curriculum, Examinations and Assessment, 2014).

- The national curriculum for physical education in Scotland focuses on developing physical competencies, cognitive skills, personal qualities and physical fitness. Outcomes and benchmarks associated with the promotion of physical activity across the key stages include: identifying and describing reasons why people participate in physical activity; sustaining energetic levels of play/activity; identifying different ways to be physically active; describing how the body changes

when active; demonstrating enthusiasm to participate; setting targets for sustaining moderate to vigorous physical activity; explaining factors that affect and influence participation; identifying types of activity where stamina is key to success; creating, implementing and monitoring personal goals for sustaining activity; and making informed choices and decisions for sustaining moderate to vigorous physical activity (Education Scotland, 2017).

- The national curriculum for physical education in Wales states that PE contributes to learners' personal and social education by prioritising activities that contribute to health, fitness and well-being throughout life. Children aged 5 to 7 years are encouraged to enjoy physical activity. Those aged 7 to 11 years begin to understand that PE involves learning how to feel healthy and stay fit while having fun; they also learn how different types of activity help them stay healthy and fit. Children aged 11 to 14 years understand that engaging in activity is beneficial to their health and fitness and take greater responsibility for their own well-being. And 14- to 16-year-olds develop a growing sense of responsibility for choosing a healthy and active lifestyle through activities that can be enjoyed and sustained both in the school and in the community (Welsh Assembly Government, 2008).

Of course, national curricula for PE undergo revisions from time to time, but the aim of promoting active lifestyles has remained prominent for decades. In fact, it has become even more central in recent times due to the trend towards a more sedentary way of life and the associated concerns about children's health (particularly the rise in childhood obesity, as outlined in chapter 1). Whilst the promotion of active lifestyles is not the only aim of PE curricula, it is a very important one; moreover, it is associated with other key aims, such as the development of movement competence.

Physical Education and Public Health

PE contributes to public health and to personal well-being through the physical learning context that it provides for every child. High-quality PE provides regular participation in physical activity, which is associated with a range of physical, psychological and social benefits (for details, see chapter 1).

In terms of young people in particular, research has found that PE can provide a number of positive outcomes, such as increased physical activity and fitness levels and improved knowledge of and attitudes towards physical activity (Bailey et al., 2009; Cale & Harris, 2006). In addition, reviews of the effects of physical activity and PE on young people's academic or cognitive performance have indicated positive (albeit weak) but positive associations; moreover, they have found no evidence that additional physical activity or PE time is detrimental to academic achievement or cognitive function (Bailey et al., 2009; Donnelly et al., 2016; Fedewa & Ahn, 2011; Keeley & Fox, 2009). One study also provides evidence that curriculum PE can provide long-term benefits. Specifically, it found that pupils who had been involved in a PE intervention 20 years earlier showed better motor fitness and reported better health and more positive attitudes towards physical activity. In addition, females who had been involved in the enhanced PE programme reported being significantly more active than their peers (Shephard & Trudeau, 2000).

From a health perspective, curriculum PE provides an inclusive learning entitlement which should ensure that all children

- are provided with opportunities to gain competence in a broad, balanced range of physical activities;
- are helped to enjoy being active and to feel confident and comfortable in a physical activity context so that they are more likely to choose to be active in their own time;
- experience and appreciate the broad range of benefits (physical, psychological and social) of a healthy, active lifestyle;
- are aware of how active they are and should be;
- know how to find and access activity opportunities in the community, including at school, around the home and in the local area; and
- understand energy balance and the need to increase physical activity in daily living in order to assist with healthy weight management.

For many young people, the school environment is a prominent source of physical activity.

For example, only 28 percent of pupils in the UK are members of an out-of-school club, and only 16 percent of girls compete in a nonschool context (Future Foundation, 2015). These statistics suggest that, for many pupils (especially girls), school PE serves as their main or only source of regular physical activity. Unfortunately, in recent decades, curriculum PE time has itself been threatened, mainly as a consequence of curriculum overcrowding and increased focus on academic attainment. As a result of this shift, some schools have squeezed PE into smaller time periods despite mounting evidence of the health benefits of physical activity for children and increasing concerns about children's health due to the trend towards sedentary living. To minimise reductions in PE time and, where necessary, to make a case for increasing it, interested persons—governors, senior staff, teaching colleagues and parents—should be informed of the health benefits of regular physical activity and the contribution that high-quality PE and extracurricular programmes make to promoting healthy, active lifestyles (Cale, Casey, & Harris, 2016).

Activity-Promoting Models and Principles in Physical Education

Active lifestyles can be promoted in PE through a range of approaches. Ideally, they sit within and make a significant contribution to a whole-school approach, as in the healthy schools and active schools models discussed in chapter 2. A schoolwide approach helps ensure that active living is advocated not just by PE teachers but by all adults in the school setting.

As part of a models-based approach to PE, a pedagogical model for **health-based physical education (HBPE)** has been proposed which takes the following as its central theme: 'pupils valuing a physically active life, so that they learn to value and practice appropriate physical activities that enhance health and well-being for the rest of their lives' (Haarens, Kirk, Cardon, & de Bourdeaudhuij, 2011, p. 330). This model requires that the affective domain (i.e., valuing physical activity) be treated prominently in planning for learning. It also calls for teachers' beliefs to be oriented towards self-actualisation and individual development in order to prepare individuals for meaningful participation in society. Thus the model prioritises both personal

THE PROMOTING ACTIVE LIFESTYLES (PAL) PROJECT

A university research team undertook an action-based study to develop and trial a principle-based approach to promoting active lifestyles that could inform policies and resources suitable for use by school PE teachers and teacher educators. The participants consisted of PE teachers and trainee teachers who were involved in an initial-teacher-training partnership and had expressed particular interest in promoting active lifestyles. Twelve participants volunteered—three teachers and nine trainee teachers—and all but one engaged with the study throughout an academic year.

Discussion points: What are the possible strengths and limitations of a principle-based approach to behaviour change? What are the pros and cons of involving both trainee teachers and experienced teachers in this study?

The participants selected and trialled principles in schools and reported back at twilight meetings every few months during the year. They also twice completed an online survey about the effects of the PAL project on pupils, themselves and their department or school. During the four meetings, the participants were introduced to and helped develop PAL principles on the whole-school and PE-specific levels; thus their voices were valued. They also discussed the implications of literature from around the world on topics related to promoting active lifestyles—for example, whole-school approaches to health, the role of fitness testing in promoting activity and health-based approaches to teaching PE.

Discussion points: What is the value of involving teachers in the development of principles? What additional health-related topics could have been included?

The meetings also provided opportunities for participants to share and discuss their experiences of trialling the principles, thus creating a supportive community of practice. Their experiences demonstrated that a principle-based approach to promoting active lifestyles can help teachers and trainee teachers alter their pedagogies to increase activity levels both within and beyond PE lessons. Participants also reported that pupils responded positively to the pedagogies.

Discussion points: What is the benefit of creating a community of practice? What limitations affected this study?

and sociocultural goals, and its subject matter is selected accordingly. The model emphasises that valuing a physically active life is a sustainable long-term process and that significant components of this process include developing knowledge and looking beyond the individual to the wider community.

Another flexible approach to promoting active lifestyles in PE is for an entire PE department to adopt PAL principles (for a whole-school PAL approach, see chapter 2). Here are some examples:

- Limit time spent getting ready before or after PE lessons; instead, maximise learning time.

- Meet the Association for Physical Education (afPE) guideline (Harris, 2015) of having pupils move for 50 percent to 80 percent of available learning time (excluding changing and getting to or from venues) by limiting the time that pupils spend receiving instructions or waiting to access equipment or resources.

- Make active use of the time spent getting to and from venues (e.g., by jogging or walking briskly) for the purpose of warming up or cooling down.

- Teach pupils about the broad range of benefits (physical, psychological and social) of a healthy, active lifestyle, including the role of physical activity in healthy weight management.

- Where appropriate, move pupils on to the next task without stopping the whole class.

- Acknowledge, praise and reward effort and progress.

- Handle assessment of learning and progress in active ways (e.g., 'show me . . .', 'demonstrate . . .', 'shadow . . .').

- Routinely inform pupils where they can be active within a few miles of the school (in every unit of work and via the school's intranet or library).

- Teach pupils how active they should be, involve them in monitoring their activity levels so they become aware of how active they are, and inform them of multiple ways to increase their activity levels.

- Identify low-activity pupils and offer them (and their parents) support, guidance and information, as well as targeted or bespoke activity sessions.

Initially, it may be prudent to adopt the principles that most PE teachers favour and consider feasible and manageable in their particular setting. Once these principles are embedded within the routine practice, additional principles can be pursued.

Health-Related Learning Outcomes

In order to promote active lifestyles, we need to establish affective, behavioural and cognitive (ABC) learning outcomes. **Affective outcomes** relate to feelings and attitudes (e.g., positive attitude towards PE), as discussed earlier in this chapter in regard to the HBPE model. **Behavioural outcomes** are associated with actions (e.g., participating in a school sport club), whereas **cognitive outcomes** involve knowledge and understanding (e.g., knowing the social health benefits of being active). Together, these types of outcomes are referred to as the ABC of health-related learning. Here are some examples of health-related ABC outcomes associated with the promotion of active lifestyles.

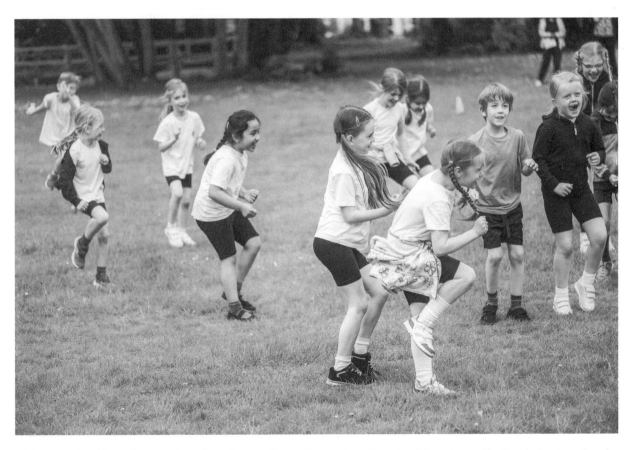

PE lessons should not focus only on keeping pupils moving; rather, they should produce affective, behavioural and cognitive learning outcomes.

Sample Health-Related ABC Outcomes for 7- to 11-Year-Olds

Pupils will do the following:

Affective

- Enjoy PE lessons.
- Look forward to being active during lunchtimes.

Behavioural

- Regularly participate in PE lessons with effort and energy.
- Choose to be active during break times.

Cognitive

- State that activity strengthens one's heart and bones.
- Describe how being active helps one feel better.

Sample Health-Related ABC Outcomes for 11- to 14-Year-Olds

Pupils will do the following:

Affective

- Feel positive about PE.
- Seek out opportunities to be active at lunchtimes.

Behavioural

- Regularly work hard to improve in PE lessons.
- Complete activity diaries that demonstrate increasing activity levels.

Cognitive

- Explain the social benefits of physical activity.
- Demonstrate the parts of a warm-up and explain their purpose.

There has been much debate about the learning associated with the promotion of active lifestyles. Back in 2000, a working group comprising representatives of national PE, sport and health organisations in England reached consensus about this learning and published health-related outcomes for children aged 5 to 16 years (Harris, 2000). These findings are presented in table 3.1, which incorporates links to relevant health-related aspects of other subjects (e.g., science; personal, social, health and economic education). To make clear the range of coverage and the progression between key stages, the learning outcomes were placed into four categories: safety issues, exercise effects, health benefits and activity promotion.

Research has indicated that outcomes related to safety issues and exercise effects are more frequently addressed by PE teachers than are outcomes associated with health benefits and activity promotion (Harris, 2009). However, the outcomes related to health benefits and activity promotion are the ones most closely linked to the promotion of active lifestyles. Therefore, we need to pay more attention to these outcomes, which have been updated to align closely with recommendations for physical activity for health (table 3.2).

Health-Related Learning Contexts

There has been much discussion about effective ways to incorporate health-related learning into physical education. One approach is to integrate the learning through the teaching of PE activity areas, such as athletics, dance, games, gymnastics, outdoor education and swimming. Another approach is to teach health-related concepts in separate units of work—for example, **health-related exercise**, **health-related fitness**, and **health and fitness**. Whilst these approaches each have their merits, they are also subject to some limitations. For example, when health-related learning is integrated through the teaching of PE activity areas, it may become lost or take second place to other learning, such as skill development and tactical understanding. Similarly, integrating health-related learning in isolated units of work may imply that it does not relate closely to the rest of the PE curriculum.

An alternative approach is to teach more-generic **health-related learning** concepts (such as those relating to safety issues and exercise effects) through all aspects of PE and to teach more-specific learning concepts (such as those associated with health benefits and activity promotion) in separate units of work. The separate units should be connected closely with curricular PE and extracurricular and community-activity programmes in order to help pupils understand that all forms of physical activity confer health benefits and can form part of a healthy lifestyle.

Research has shown that PE teachers generally accept their responsibility to promote active lifestyles and that the majority articulate a 'fit-

TABLE 3.1 Health-Related Learning Outcomes for Ages 5 to 16

Pupils who are 5 to 7 years old can do the following:

Safety issues	• Identify and adhere to safety rules and practices (e.g., changing clothes for PE lessons; tying long hair back; not wearing jewellery; sitting and standing with good posture; wearing footwear when skipping with a rope; not running fast to touch walls). • Explain that activity starts with a gentle warm-up and finishes with a calming cool-down.
Exercise effects	• Recognise, describe and feel the effects of exercise, including changes to • breathing (e.g., it becomes faster and deeper), • heart rate (e.g., heart pumps faster), • temperature (e.g., person feels hotter), • appearance (e.g., person looks hotter), • feelings (e.g., person feels good, more energetic, tired) and • external body parts (e.g., arm and leg muscles are working). • Explain that the body uses food and drink to release energy for exercise.
Health benefits	• Explain that regular exercise improves health by • helping one feel good (e.g., happy, pleased, content) and helping body parts (e.g., bones, muscles) grow, develop and work well.
Activity promotion	• Identify when, where and how they can be active at school (both in and out of lessons). • Use opportunities to be active, including at playtimes.

Pupils who are 7 to 11 years old can do the following:

Safety issues	• Explain the need for safety rules and practices (e.g., adopting good posture at all times; being hygienic; changing clothes and having a wash after energetic activity; wearing footwear as appropriate; following rules; protecting against cold weather; avoiding sunburn; lifting safely; using space sensibly [not bumping into others]). • Identify the purpose of warming up and cooling down and recognise and describe the parts of a warm-up and of a cool-down: exercises for the joints (e.g., arm circles), whole-body activities (e.g., jogging, skipping without a rope) and stretches for either the whole body (e.g., reaching long and tall) or parts of the body (e.g., lower-leg or calf muscles).
Exercise effects	• Explain and feel the short-term effects of exercise. • Breathing rate and depth increase to provide more oxygen to working muscles. • Heart rate increases to pump more oxygen to working muscles. • Temperature increases because working muscles produce energy in the form of heat; as that heat is transferred to the body's surface (skin) to control body temperature, the skin can become moist, sticky and sweaty. • Appearance can become flushed due to blood vessels widening and getting closer to the surface of the skin. • Feelings and moods can vary (e.g., having fun, feeling good among friends). • Explain that the body needs a certain amount of energy every day in the form of food and drink in order to function properly (e.g., for normal growth, development and daily living) and that body fat increases if more calories are taken in than are needed (e.g., for breathing, growing, sleeping, eating, moving, exercising).
Health benefits	• Explain that exercise strengthens bones and muscles (including the heart) and helps keep joints flexible. Explain that exercise can help one feel good about oneself and can be fun and social (e.g., involves sharing experiences and cooperating with others). • Explain that regular exercise improves one's physical capacity and therefore permits daily activities to be performed more easily. • Explain that being active helps one maintain a healthy body weight.
Activity promotion	• Monitor their current levels of activity (e.g., daily, twice weekly). • Identify when, where and how they can be active, both in and outside of school. • Make decisions about which physical activities they enjoy and explain that individuals have different feelings about the types and amounts of activity they do. • Use opportunities to be active for 30 to 60 minutes every day (with rest periods as necessary), including lessons, playtimes and club activities.

(continued)

Table 3.1 (continued)

Pupils who are 11 to 14 years old can do the following:

Safety issues	• Demonstrate their understanding of safe exercise practices (e.g., tying long hair back and removing jewellery to avoid injury; adopting good posture when sitting, standing or moving; performing exercises with good technique; having a wash or shower following energetic activity; using equipment and facilities with permission and, where necessary, under supervision; administering basic first aid; wearing adequate protection, such as goalkeeping gloves and leg pads, as appropriate; coping with specific weather conditions, such as using sunscreen to avoid sunburn and drinking fluids to prevent dehydration; following proper procedures for specific activities). • Demonstrate their concern for and understanding of back care by lifting, carrying, placing and using equipment responsibly and with good technique. • Explain why certain exercises and practices are not recommended (e.g., standing toe touches, straight-leg sit-ups, bounces during stretching, flinging movements) and be able to perform safe alternatives (e.g., sit-and-reach stretch, curl-up with bent legs, stretches held still, movements performed with control). • Explain the value of purposefully preparing for and recovering from activity and the possible consequences of not doing so. • More specifically, explain the purpose of, and plan and perform, each component of a warm-up and of a cool-down (i.e., mobility exercises, whole-body activities, static stretches) both for activity in general (e.g., games, athletics) and for specific activities (e.g., volleyball, high jump, circuit training). • Use good technique in performing developmentally appropriate cardiorespiratory activities, as well as strength and flexibility exercises, for each major muscle group.

Exercise effects	• Explain and monitor a range of short-term effects of exercise on
	  • the cardiovascular system (e.g., changes in breathing, heart rate, temperature, appearance, feelings, recovery rate and ability to pace oneself and remain within a target zone) and
	  • the musculoskeletal system (e.g., increases in muscular strength, endurance and flexibility; improved muscle tone and posture; enhanced functional capacity and sport or dance performance).
	• Explain that appropriate training can improve fitness and performance and that specific types of activity affect specific aspects of fitness (e.g., running affects cardiorespiratory fitness)
	• Explain the differences between whole-body activities (e.g., walking, jogging, cycling, dancing, swimming) that help reduce body fat and conditioning exercises (e.g., straight and twisting curl-ups) that improve muscle tone.

Health benefits	• Explain a range of long-term benefits of exercise for physical health, such as
	  • reduced risk of chronic disease (e.g., heart disease),
	  • reduced risk of bone disease (e.g., osteoporosis),
	  • reduced risk of some other health conditions (e.g., obesity, back pain) and
	  • improved management of some health conditions (e.g., asthma, diabetes, arthritis).
	• Explain that exercise can enhance mental health and social and psychological well-being (e.g., enjoyment of being with friends; increased confidence and self-esteem; decreased anxiety and stress) and that an appropriate balance between work, leisure and exercise promotes good health.
	• Explain that increasing activity levels and eating a balanced diet can help one maintain a healthy body weight (i.e., energy balance), that the body needs at least a certain minimum intake of daily energy in order to function properly and that strict dieting and excessive exercising can damage one's health.
	• Explain how each activity area (athletics, dance, games, gymnastics, swimming and outdoor and adventurous activities) can contribute to physical health and to social and psychological well-being (e.g., can improve stamina, assist in weight management, strengthen bones, be enjoyable).

Activity promotion	• Access information about a range of activity opportunities at school, at home and in the local community and identify ways to incorporate activity into their lifestyles (e.g., walking or cycling to school or to meet friends; helping around the home or garden). • Reflect on their activity strengths and preferences and know how to get involved in activities. • Participate in activity of at least moderate intensity for a minimum of half an hour and preferably for one hour every day (i.e., 30 to 60 minutes accumulated over the course of the day). • Participate at least twice a week in activities (e.g., dance, aerobics, skipping, games, body conditioning, resistance exercises) that enhance or help maintain muscular strength and flexibility, as well as bone health. • Monitor and evaluate personal activity levels over a period of time (e.g., by keeping an activity diary for four to six weeks and reflecting on the experience).

Pupils who are 14 to 16 years old can do the following:

Safety issues	• Recognise and manage risk and apply safe exercise principles and procedures (e.g., not exercising when unwell or injured; avoiding prolonged high-impact exercise; administering first aid, including resuscitation techniques; avoiding excessive amounts of exercise). • Evaluate warm-ups and cool-downs in terms of safety, effectiveness and relevance to the specific activity and take responsibility for their own safe and effective preparation for and recovery from activity. • Select, perform and evaluate exercises from a range of lifetime activities (e.g., jogging, swimming, cycling, aerobics, step aerobics, circuit training, weight training) with an eye toward safety, effectiveness and developmental appropriateness.
Exercise effects	• Explain that training and practice affect performance and are activity specific. • Explain that training programmes develop both health-related components of physical and mental fitness (cardiorespiratory fitness, muscular strength and endurance, flexibility, body composition, composure and decision making) and skill-related components (agility, balance, coordination, power, reaction time, speed, concentration and determination).
Health benefits	• Explain that frequent and appropriate exercise enhances the physical, social and psychological well-being of all individuals, regardless of age, able-bodiedness or disability, and the presence or absence of health conditions (e.g., asthma, depression) and chronic disease (e.g., arthritis). • Explain that exercise can help one manage stress and contribute to a happy, healthy and balanced lifestyle. • Appreciate the risks associated with a sedentary lifestyle and with excessive behaviour (e.g., overexercising, disordered eating). • Identify how each activity area (e.g., gymnastics, swimming, athletics) can contribute to specific components of health-related fitness; for example, gymnastics involves weight-bearing actions and thus develops muscular strength and endurance.
Activity promotion	• Plan, perform, monitor and evaluate a safe and effective health-related exercise programme that meets their personal needs and preferences over an extended period of time (e.g., 6 to 12 weeks). • Access physical activity personnel (e.g., sport development officers, active school coordinators, coaches, instructors), facilities (e.g., leisure centres; sport, health and fitness clubs) and services (e.g., courses, projects, leaflets, pamphlets) in the local community. • Demonstrate a range of lifetime physical activities (e.g., walking, jogging, swimming, cycling, aerobics, step aerobics, circuit training, weight training, skipping, aqua exercise). • Explain and demonstrate practical understanding of the key principles of exercise programming and training, including • progression (developing the amount of exercise by gradually increasing frequency, intensity, duration or a combination of these factors); • overload (progressively enabling the body to do more exercise than accustomed to); • specificity (doing a particular exercise or sporting activity to benefit specific muscles, joints, bones and energy systems); • balance, moderation and variety (maximising exercise benefits and minimising risks); • maintenance (establishing a routine, sustaining a commitment and coping with relapse); • reversibility (gradually losing the benefits of exercise if it is discontinued); and • cost–benefit ratio (weighing costs such as time, money, transport and sweat against benefits such as maintaining body weight, feeling good and improving health and fitness). • Assess their own qualities, skills, achievements and potential so that they can set personal goals that help them follow the activity recommendations for young people and develop a commitment to an active lifestyle. • Explain constraints on being active and explore how to overcome them in order to access and sustain involvement in activity.

Adapted, by permission, from J. Harris, 2000, *Health-related exercise in the National Curriculum. Key stages 1 to 4* (Leeds: Human Kinetics).

TABLE 3.2   Learning Outcomes That Promote Health and Activity for Ages 5 to 16

Pupils who are 5 to 7 years old can do the following:

Health benefits	• Explain that regular activity improves health by
	  • helping one feel good (e.g., happy, pleased, content) and
	  • helping body parts (e.g., bones and muscles) grow, develop and work well.

Activity Promotion	• Identify when, where and how they can be active at school (in and out of lessons). • Use opportunities to be active, including at playtimes.

Pupils who are 7 to 11 years old can do the following:

Health benefits	• Explain that activity strengthens bones and muscles (including the heart) and helps keep joints flexible. • Explain that activity can help one feel good about oneself and can be fun and social (e.g., sharing experiences and cooperating with others). • Explain that regular activity permits one to perform daily activities more easily. • Explain that being active helps one maintain a healthy body weight.
Activity Promotion	• Monitor their current levels of activity (e.g., daily, twice weekly). • Identify when, where and how they can be active in and outside of school. • Make decisions about which physical activities they enjoy and explain that individuals have different feelings about the types and amounts of activity to do. • Use opportunities to be active for one hour per day (with rest periods as necessary), including lessons, playtimes and club activities.

Pupils who are 11 to 14 years old can do the following:

Health benefits	• Explain a range of long-term benefits of activity for physical health, including
	  • reduced risk of chronic disease (e.g., heart disease),
	  • reduced risk of bone disease (e.g., osteoporosis),
	  • reduced risk of some other health conditions (e.g., obesity, back pain) and
	  • improved management of some health conditions (e.g., asthma, diabetes).
	• Explain that activity can enhance mental health and social and psychological well-being (e.g., enjoying being with friends, increased confidence and self-esteem, decreased anxiety and stress) and that an appropriate balance between work, leisure and activity promotes good health.
	• Explain that increasing activity levels and eating a balanced diet can help maintain a healthy body weight (energy balance), that the body needs at least a certain minimum intake of daily energy in order to function properly, and that strict dieting and excessive exercising can damage one's health.
	• Explain how each activity area (athletics, dance, games, gymnastics, swimming and outdoor and adventurous activities) can contribute to physical health and to social and psychological well-being (e.g., can improve stamina, assist in weight management, strengthen bones, be enjoyable).

Activity Promotion	• Access information about a range of activity opportunities at school, at home and in the local community and identify ways to incorporate activity into their lifestyles (e.g., walking or cycling to school or to meet friends; helping around the home or garden). • Reflect on their activity strengths and preferences and know how to go about getting involved in activities. • Participate in activity of at least moderate intensity for one hour every day (accumulated over the course of the day), including activity that strengthens muscles and bones. • Monitor and evaluate personal activity levels over a period of time (e.g., by keeping an activity diary for four to six weeks and reflecting on the experience).

Pupils who are 14 to 16 years old can do the following:

Health benefits	• Explain that frequent and appropriate activity enhances the physical, social and psychological well-being of all individuals, regardless of age, able-bodiedness or disability, and the presence or absence of health conditions (e.g., asthma, depression) and chronic disease (e.g., arthritis). • Explain that activity can help one manage stress and contribute to a happy, healthy and balanced lifestyle. • Appreciate the risks associated with a sedentary lifestyle and with excessive behaviour (e.g., overexercising, disordered eating). • Identify how each activity area (e.g., gymnastics, swimming, athletics) can contribute to specific components of health-related fitness; for example, gymnastics involves weight-bearing actions and thus develops muscular strength and endurance.

Activity Promotion	• Plan, perform, monitor and evaluate a safe and effective activity programme that meets their personal needs and preferences over an extended period of time (e.g., 6 to 12 weeks) and meets the guidelines for physical activity for health.
	• Access physical activity personnel (e.g., sport development officers, coaches, instructors), facilities (e.g., leisure centres; sport, health and fitness clubs) and services (e.g., courses, projects, leaflets, pamphlets) in the local community.
	• Demonstrate a range of lifetime physical activities (e.g., walking, jogging, swimming, cycling, aerobics, step aerobics, circuit training, weight training, skipping, aqua activity).
	• Explain and demonstrate practical understanding of the key principles of activity programming and training, including
	  • progression (developing the amount of activity by gradually increasing frequency, intensity, duration, or a combination of these factors),
	  • overload (progressively enabling the body to do more activity than previously accustomed to),
	  • specificity (doing a particular exercise or sporting activity to benefit specific muscles, joints, bones and energy systems),
	  • balance, moderation and variety (maximising activity benefits and minimising risks),
	  • maintenance (establishing a routine, sustaining a commitment and coping with relapse),
	  • reversibility (gradually losing the benefits of exercise if it is discontinued) and
	  • cost–benefit ratio (weighing costs such as time, money, transport and sweat against benefits such as maintaining body weight, feeling good and improving health and fitness).
	• Assess their own qualities, skills, achievements and potential so that they can set personal goals that help them follow the activity recommendations for young people and develop a commitment to an active lifestyle.
	• Explain constraints on being active and explore how to overcome them in order to access and sustain involvement in activity.

Adapted, by permission, from J. Harris, 2000, *Health-related exercise in the National Curriculum. Key stages 1 to 4* (Leeds: Human Kinetics).

ness for life' philosophy focused on the role of physical activity in maintaining and enhancing health (Harris & Leggett, 2015a, 2015b). Their teaching *practices*, however, have been found to generally reflect a 'fitness for performance' philosophy focused on the role of physical activity in developing and increasing fitness. Characteristics of these two philosophies are presented in table 3.3 (Harris & Leggett, 2015a, 2015b).

It has been suggested that this curious mismatch between articulated philosophy (fitness for life) and practice (fitness for performance) may be influenced by the following factors: PE teachers' sporting backgrounds, the fact that their university and teacher-training courses are typically oriented towards sport science, and their limited awareness of and exposure to fitness-for-life pedagogies (Harris & Leggett, 2015a, 2015b). Whatever its cause, the gap between health-related rhetoric and practice has led to calls for critical pedagogies, known as 'PE for health', that take a sociocultural and evidence-based approach (Armour & Harris, 2013; Burrows, Wright, & McCormack, 2009). Such pedagogies are reflected and exemplified in parts 2 and 3 of this book.

TABLE 3.3   Characteristics of Fitness-for-Life and Fitness-for-Performance Approaches in Physical Education

	Fitness for life	Fitness for performance
Sources and influences	Primary and public health	Sport science and biomedicine
Dominant foci	Role of physical activity in maintaining or enhancing health	Role of physical activity in developing or increasing fitness
	Desire for pupils to be fit enough to undertake and enjoy everyday activities	Desire for pupils to be fit for sport
	Promotion of active lifestyles	Emphasis on improving sport performance
	Focus on participation	Emphasis on fitness testing and training and on conditioning activities linked to sport performance
	Broad PE curriculum including lifetime activities	Limited PE curriculum dominated by competitive games and fitness-related activities
	Freedom for older pupils (14- to 16-year-olds) to choose their activities	Freedom for pupils to design sport-related training programmes based on fitness components and training principles
	Focus on helping pupils become increasingly independent in being active, both at school and beyond	
	Focus on recreational activities in extracurricular programmes	
	Activity monitoring associated with recommended levels of physical activity for young people	

Assessment of Health-Related Learning

Health-related learning can be assessed through written, verbal and active responses to questions, tasks and tests. More specifically, affective and behavioural outcomes can be assessed by means of teacher observation of effort and commitment in PE lessons, participation records for PE lessons and extracurricular activities, and activity monitoring (e.g., activity diaries) and fitness testing. Cognitive outcomes, on the other hand, can be assessed through question-and-answer episodes (e.g., addressing the benefits of being active) and through practical and active tasks (e.g., demonstrating a range of aerobic activities, performing exercises to strengthen or stretch particular muscle groups). The web resource for this chapter includes two sample assessments that you may use or modify to suit your needs.

Peer- and self-assessment are particularly appropriate for health-related learning as they directly involve pupils in making judgements and decisions about their own learning and that

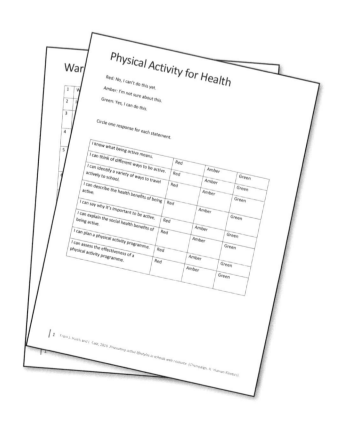

of their peers, which helps them take ownership of their health. Active assessment tasks are also encouraged, as they help increase pupils' activity levels in PE lessons. Here are some examples of methods for assessing health-related learning:

Focused Questions

- How do you feel when you are active?
- What happens to your breathing when you exercise?
- Why does your heart rate change when you exercise?
- Which muscles are working hard when you run?
- What is one reason that being active is good for your health? What else can you say about that? What is another reason? (Continue prompting to ensure inclusion of physical, psychological and social health benefits.)
- Talk to a partner about how being active helps you maintain a healthy weight. (Ask for volunteers to share their ideas with another group or with the whole class, or ask specific pairs or pupils for their responses.)
- Why is it important to stretch muscles after you have worked them hard?
- How much activity should young people do?
- Explain to a partner how stronger upper-body muscles help you throw further.
- What are some of the main reasons that some young people are not active?

Practical Tasks

- Show me an exercise that makes your heart pump faster.
- Demonstrate a stretch for the muscles in the back of your leg.
- Perform an exercise that strengthens your tummy (stomach or abdominal) muscles.
- With a partner, design a warm-up for the long jump; include activities to mobilise joints in the legs and to warm your major leg muscles, followed by stretches of the main muscles used in jumping.
- Observe another group's cool-down for sprinting and decide how effective it is in reducing heart and breathing rates and stretching out the main muscles that are worked hard when sprinting.

- For next week's lesson, make a list of places in the local area where you can be active (other than at school).
- Keep an activity diary for one school day; include in it all activity that you do, such as walking, cycling or scooting to and from school; being active at breaks or lunchtimes; playing sport, exercising or dancing in school or outside of school; and performing any active jobs you do at home, such as cleaning, gardening or going to and from the shops. Add up all the minutes of activity you have done in one day. Does it amount to at least 60 minutes (one hour) of activity?

Health-Related Learning Support

A wealth of support for health-related learning is available from numerous associations and organisations, including national PE, health and sport bodies. This support takes the form of programmes, resources and professional development opportunities associated with participation in physical activity.

For example, the Association for Physical Education (afPE) is the only physical-education subject association in the United Kingdom, and its purpose is to promote and maintain high standards and safe practice in all aspects and at all levels of PE. To meet this purpose, it seeks to influence developments at both national and local events, in part by working to raise awareness of PE's contributions to public health and well-being. It pursues this objective by providing information on its website; in its professional journal, *Physical Education Matters* (e.g., its position statement on health [Harris, 2015] and its perspectives on fitness testing); at conferences and events; through professional learning opportunities; and through its contributions to national campaigns, such as Sport England's This Girl Can, in the form of resources for schools.

In another example, the Association for Young People's Health supports evidence-based practices in adolescent health and health care. It also works on a range of initiatives to increase young people's voice and involvement in decisions that affect their health and works with a range of professionals to improve health services for young people. Every two years, it publishes key data on adolescence, including information about lifestyle and

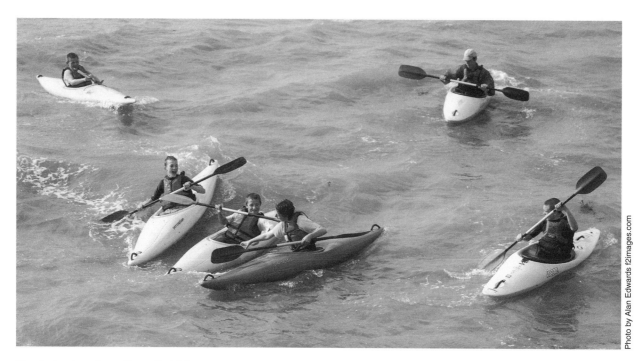

Physical education offers all children opportunities to access the outdoor environment and to learn about themselves through fun, exciting challenges and adventures

health-related behaviours (Association for Young People's Health, 2017).

SSEHS Active (http://www.ssehsactive.org.uk/) is part of the School of Sport, Exercise and Health Sciences at Loughborough University. The School is a key partner of the National Centre for Sport and Exercise Medicine. SSEHS Active aims to develop, translate and disseminate research and practice-based evidence to expand and improve effective practice of physical activity promotion in the UK. Its website includes high quality resources for practitioners, some of which emanated from the previous British Heart Foundation National Centre for Physical Activity and Health based at Loughborough. Examples of resources on the website include: a booklet titled 'Interpreting the UK physical activity guidelines for children' which helps adults working with children and young people (e.g. teachers, parents, youth workers) to use the Government's physical activity guidelines; and report cards which give information about the physical activity of children and youth across a number of countries, including England, Scotland and Wales. The website also provides a comprehensive informa-

tion service on physical activity news, events and publications as well as details of ongoing projects such as the 'CLASS PAL' which works with schools to develop, implement and evaluate a 'toolbox' of strategies for teachers to use to break up or reduce the sitting time of primary school pupils in the classroom (which helps facilitate a whole school approach to activity, as encouraged in chapter 2).

Sport England, Sport Northern Ireland, Sport Scotland and Sport Wales all have a remit to promote participation in physical activity and have developed campaigns, programmes and projects involving school-age children and young people. For example, Sport England has devised the national campaign This Girl Can to get girls and women moving regardless of shape, size or ability, as well as the Sportivate project to give more young people the chance to discover a sport that they love. Sport Northern Ireland launched the Activ8 campaign to raise awareness among children and young people of the importance of taking part in at least 60 minutes of physical activity every day and of eating a healthy and balanced diet (as mentioned in chapter 1). Sport Scotland created an Active Schools programme to encourage children and young people to get active and stay active, as well as an Active Girls initiative to increase girls' and young women's participation in PE, sport and physical activity through programmes such as: YDance Active, Active Girls, and Fit for Girls. Sport Wales is also involved in a number of programmes in schools, such as Play to Learn, Dragon Multi-Skills & Sport, and Physical Literacy 5×60.

The Youth Sport Trust (YST) is an independent charity devoted to changing young people's lives by helping them achieve their full potential through high-quality PE and sport opportunities. The YST provides resources and professional learning events and supports schools' efforts to enhance their pupils' achievements and aspirations. Particular examples among many include their work with schools on the My Personal Best programme, which is associated with character development through PE, Start to Move, Active Kids and their support of 'innovation and lead schools' that focus on a range of specialisms, including health and well-being.

Additional sources of information include government departments of education and health, as well as associated organisations, such as Public Health England, Public Health Wales, the Scottish Public Health Network, and Public Health Agency in Northern Ireland. The latter, for example, has produced an activity-record booklet (It All Adds Up) to help young children track their amount of physical activity. Numerous other resources to help teachers promote healthy, active lifestyles are available from subject associations and organisations such as the PSHE Association (i.e., the association for personal, social, health and economic education) in England and the Social, Personal and Health Education (SPHE) Support Service in Scotland.

Summary

The promotion of active lifestyles has become an increasingly prominent aim of PE curricula around the world due to the trend towards a more sedentary way of life and associated concerns about children's health. As a result, governors, senior staff, teaching colleagues and parents should be aware of the range of health benefits provided by regular physical activity and the contribution that high-quality PE and extracurricular programmes make to promoting healthy, active lifestyles.

The promotion of active lifestyles within PE can be approached in a variety of ways, such as adopting a specific health-based model or activity-enhancing principles to attain health-related learning outcomes in the affective, behavioural and cognitive domains. Health-related learning can be taught through all aspects of PE, as well as in discrete units of work that make close connections with curricular PE and extracurricular and community-activity programmes. However, teachers should be aware of the common mismatch between a fitness-for-life philosophy, on one hand, and, on the other hand, teaching practices that reflect a philosophy of fitness for performance. To resolve this gap, teachers should seek to adopt 'PE for health' pedagogies that are critical, sociocultural and evidence based. Health-related learning can be assessed via a wide range of methods, among which peer assessment, self-assessment and active assessment are particularly appropriate. A wealth of health-related learning support is available for teachers in the form of programmes, resources and professional development opportunities associated with participation in physical activity.

PART II

Monitoring Health, Activity and Fitness in Schools

Monitoring Health in Schools

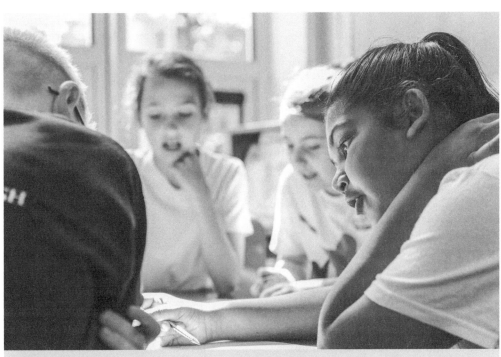

Chapter Objectives

After reading this chapter, you will be able to

- ▶ recognise health definitions, behaviours and descriptors;
- ▶ understand the rationale for monitoring children's health;
- ▶ identify methods for monitoring children's health in schools;
- ▶ describe key findings from some school-based child measurement programmes;
- ▶ promote learning through monitoring children's health and
- ▶ implement practical ideas and tools for monitoring children's health.

This chapter considers the rationale for the increased prominence given to monitoring children's health in schools. It also describes and critiques school-based national child measurement programmes in the United Kingdom; more specifically, it reports key findings from these programmes and outlines alternative forms of health monitoring that focus on adopting healthy, active lifestyles. In a school setting, children's health behaviours can be monitored using child-friendly questionnaires and diaries, and this chapter describes pedagogically appropriate examples that can help you implement effective health monitoring within the curriculum.

Defining Health

Health was initially defined by the World Health Organisation (WHO) not merely as the absence of disease or infirmity but as a state of complete physical, mental and social well-being (WHO, 1948). This definition was later expanded to describe health as a resource for everyday life and a positive concept emphasising social and personal resources, as well as physical capacities (WHO, 1986). These definitions demonstrate the multidimensional nature of health (physical, mental and social) and its complex relationship with everyday living. However, despite their usefulness in outlining the parameters of health, they are problematic to operationalise. Specifically, it is difficult to use them to assess one's own state of health or to determine someone else's health status. For example, what does a 'state of complete physical, mental and social well-being' feel like? What 'social and personal resources' are required, and how much of them is necessary to be in 'good health'?

Consequently, practitioners tend to turn to descriptors of health behaviours to help learners understand what it means to lead a healthy lifestyle. For example, positive health behaviours might include the following:

- Eating a balanced diet, including fruits and vegetables
- Drinking plenty of water every day
- Getting sufficient sleep
- Maintaining a sensible balance between work, rest and play (or relaxation)
- Not smoking

- Drinking alcohol in moderation or not at all
- Remaining in control of one's emotions
- Coping with the day-to-day pressures and stresses of work
- Being active every day
- Feeling happy

These descriptors can be used to trigger discussions among children about their own lifestyles and what, if anything, could be changed to improve their health status. In this vein, the web resource for this chapter includes case studies of three young people (see the document titled Examples of Young People's Lifestyles) that can be used to generate discussion among children. Here are some possible starter questions:

- How healthy is this person?
- What, if anything, could this person do to improve his or her health?
- What might help the person do so?
- What might prevent the person from doing so?

Children can also be encouraged to write a short narrative, profile or blog paragraph about their own lifestyle (similar to the examples provided in the web resource). These responses can be used anonymously to discuss what it means

---

Examples of Young People's Lifestyles

Sam

Sam is 16 years old and a keen sportsperson; specifically, she is a member of a local football club and a tennis club. An outgoing and sociable person, she enjoys her PE lessons and is considering teaching PE as a career. Sam is slim and generally eats what she wants; she particularly enjoys fast food. She drinks alcohol in moderation at weekends and has the occasional cigarette when she is out with friends. She is generally happy and optimistic.

Chris

Chris is 14 years old and generally dislikes PE and most sports; he takes part in school PE lessons but shows little enthusiasm. On the other hand, he cycles to school each day and enjoys skateboarding at weekends. He tends to be a loner and spends much of his free time alone in his bedroom, watching TV, listening to loud music and using his computer. He is a little overweight and enjoys his food. He does not drink alcohol and does not smoke. He is a bit of a worrier and can feel down at times.

Jo

Jo is 13 years old. She willingly takes part in PE lessons and is a reserve for the school netball team. She would like to join a club outside of school but doesn't think she's good enough. She has the same small circle of friends inside and outside of school, and they enjoy talking, shopping and going to the cinema. Jo is neither overweight nor slim. She is a 'fussy' eater who eats lots of fruit but hates vegetables. Jo has drunk cider at the occasional party and tried a cigarette once but didn't enjoy it. In terms of moods, she has highs and lows.

to be healthy, how health is affected by factors both within and beyond an individual's control, and what can be achieved collectively and individually to improve public health. You are encouraged to be creative both in your methods of monitoring pupils' health and in the ways in which you use the information gathered. See the following case study for one school's approach to monitoring health behaviours and promoting positive ones.

Health descriptors can be further developed to include specific public health recommendations for children and young people. For example, the 'being active every day' descriptor can be replaced with a more precise descriptor, such as 'being active for at least one hour per day' or 'accumulating at least 60 minutes per day of moderate- to vigorous-intensity physical activity'. Health behaviour questionnaires that use specific public health recommendations are presented in the web resource for this chapter.

How Healthy Are You? (Primary Ages)

Being healthy	Always	Sometimes	Never
Do you eat fruits and vegetables every day?			
Do you drink water every day?			
Do you have plenty of sleep each night?			
Do you feel happy?			
Are you active for about an hour every day?			

1 From I. Harris and L. Cale, 2019, *Promoting active lifestyles in schools web resource*. (Champaign, IL: Human Kinetics).

HEALTHY HOMEWORK INITIATIVE

One primary school in the East Midlands introduced a Healthy Homework initiative as a way to promote positive health behaviours among its pupils beyond the school gates. At the start of the school term, all pupils were given a Healthy Homework journal and bag (containing a ball, a skipping rope, a soft bat, a beanbag and a cone) and encouraged to participate in healthy behaviours outside of school. Examples of such behaviours included choosing healthy food and drink options at home (e.g., fruits, vegetables, no- or low-sugar drinks) and being active (e.g., walking, cycling or scooting to and from school or shops; taking part in physical activity sessions and sport clubs).

Discussion points: What are the possible advantages and disadvantages of packaging healthy behaviours as homework? What are your thoughts about the content of the Healthy Homework bag?

Pupils were encouraged to record their healthy behaviours in their journal on a daily basis, and parents were asked to sign the journal at the end of each week. The journals were used by class teachers to prompt discussion with pupils about the consequences of healthy and unhealthy behaviours. The initiative was evaluated after one term. The vast majority of the younger pupils (8- and 9-year-olds) had enthusiastically engaged with the initiative, completed their Healthy Homework journals each week and made good use of the items in their Healthy Homework bags. Engagement was lower, however, among older pupils (9- and 10-year-olds); in fact, about a quarter of those pupils no longer recorded healthy behaviours after a few weeks unless prompted to do so by their class teachers.

Discussion points: Why do you think the older pupils were less engaged with the initiative? How might their engagement be increased?

Despite these mixed results, responses were generally positive from most of the teachers and from many parents, although about a third of parents had not signed the journals on a weekly basis. The school plans to discuss the findings of the evaluation with school governors and parent groups and then improve the initiative for future years.

Discussion points: What might be done to increase the proportion of parents who sign the journals? How might the initiative as a whole be improved for future years?

Rationale for Monitoring Children's Health

Monitoring children's health is considered important both because cardiovascular disease has its origins in childhood and because obesity rates are increasing among children and are associated with health conditions such as type 2 diabetes. The emphasis on monitoring also derives in part from growing concerns about children's mental health, given that 20 percent of children experience mental health problems and 10 percent have a clinically diagnosable mental health disorder (World Health Organisation, 2005). More specifically, the United Kingdom ranked last among 21 of the world's richest countries in UNICEF's report on children's well-being in 2007, 16th out of 29 in 2013 and 20th out of 35 of the world's richest countries in 2016 (United Nations Children's Fund, 2007, 2013, 2016).

The rationale for monitoring children's health is strengthened by the fact that patterns of health-related behaviours are often acquired and established during childhood; therefore, helping children become aware of their health status constitutes an important aspect of behaviour change. With this end in mind, it is prudent to undertake some health monitoring in schools, which reach virtually all children and hold the potential to improve the health of young people (and their families) by providing professionally delivered programmes and services that promote healthy lifestyles. Of course, schools are limited in the extent to which they can monitor children's health, as they do not have the expertise, time or funding to undertake precise, comprehensive measurements of, for example, blood pressure, blood lipids or depression. However, they may feel able to make use of low-cost, noninvasive methods of exploring health outcomes and behaviours, such as eating and activity habits and general level of satisfaction with school and life.

Methods of Monitoring Children's Health

In some countries, including England and Wales, government departments have established school-based national child measurement programmes to do the following:

- Tackle obesity.

- Gather population-level data to allow analysis of trends in growth patterns and obesity.
- Inform local planning and delivery of services for children.
- Increase public and professional understanding of weight issues in children and serve as a vehicle for engaging with children and families about healthy lifestyles.

As part of these programmes in England and Wales, the heights and weights of children aged 4 or 5 years (in Wales) plus those aged 10 or 11 years (in England) are measured and used to calculate their body mass index (BMI). Specifically, BMI is the quotient of weight (expressed in kilograms) divided by the square of height (expressed in metres). Written feedback about children's weight status is provided to their parents. Participation is not compulsory, but nonparticipation is handled on an opt-out basis only.

Operational guidance about how to undertake the measuring is provided by organisations such as Public Health England, which states the following:

- Ensure that parents receive a letter explaining the purpose of the programme and provide them with the opportunity to withdraw their child from it.
- Aim to provide results to parents within six weeks of measurement.
- The privacy and dignity of the child must be safeguarded at all times, and the measurement is to be done sensitively in a private setting.
- Height and weight information must be gathered by health professionals with minimal physical contact.
- Individual children's results will not be shared with school staff or other pupils, and suppression and disclosure controls will be implemented when the data set and publication are released to ensure that individual children cannot be identified.

Based on National Health Service (NHS) Digital, 2016.

Key Findings of National Child Measurement Programmes

For the 2015–2016 year, the National Child Measurement Programme in England was based on more than a million measurements of children in

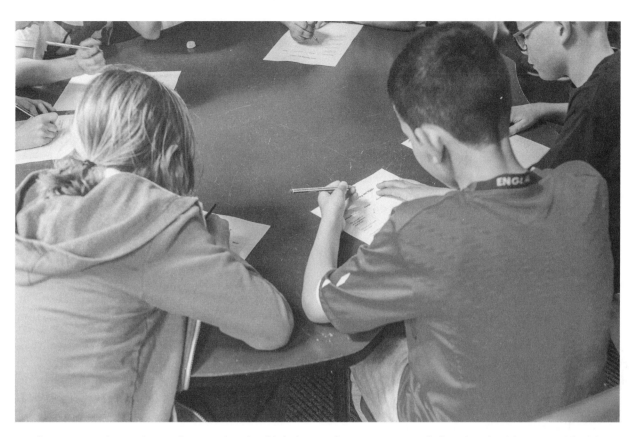

Teachers can guide pupils to reflect on their health habits and to set targets to help adopt healthy, active lifestyles.

state-maintained schools, representing some 95 percent of those eligible. Key findings included the following:

- The prevalence of obese 4- and 5-year-old children (9.3 percent) was higher than in 2014–2015 (9.1 percent) but lower than in 2006–2007 (9.9 percent). The prevalence of obese 10- and 11-year-old children was higher (19.8 percent) than in 2014–2015 (19.1 percent) and 2006–2007 (17.5 percent).

- More than a fifth (22.1 percent) of 4- and 5-year-old children were either overweight or obese, which was higher than in 2014–2015 (21.9 percent) but slightly lower than in 2006–2007 (22.9 percent). Approximately one-third (34.2 percent) of 10- and 11-year-old children were either overweight or obese, which was higher than in 2014–2015 (33.2 percent) and 2006-2007 (31.6 percent).

- Obesity prevalence for children living in the most deprived areas was double that of those living in the least deprived areas. Specifically, obesity prevalence among 4- and 5-year-old children living in the most deprived areas was 12.5 percent, as compared with 5.5 percent among those living in the least deprived areas. For 10- and 11-year-old children, the figures were 26 percent and 11.7 percent, respectively.

- Obesity prevalence varied by local authority—for example, ranging from 11 percent to 28.5 percent for 10- and 11-year-old children living in London boroughs.

Based on Public Health Wales National Health Services (NHS) Trust, 2017.

The Child Measurement Programme for Wales only involved children aged 4 or 5 years during the 2015–2016 academic year. Key findings included the following:

- Participation rates fell to 93.3 percent in 2015–2016 from 94.5 percent in 2014–2015. In terms of sheer numbers, over 33,000 children's measurements were included in 2015-2016.

- Nearly three-quarters (72.9 percent) of the children measured had a BMI classified as healthy, the same proportion as in the previous year.

- The prevalence of 4- to 5-year-old children found to be obese in Wales (11.7 percent) was significantly higher than in England (9.3 percent). It was also significantly higher in Wales than in any of the individual English regions, where the highest prevalence was 10.7 percent (in North East England).

- A strong relationship was found between levels of obesity and deprivation; specifically, 13.5 percent of children in the most deprived areas were obese, as compared with 8.8 percent in the least deprived areas.

Public Health Wales National Health Service [NHS] Trust, 2017.

Critique of National Child Health Measurement Programmes

Whilst population-level information about children may have its uses, child health measurement programmes such as those just described are controversial. For one thing, they are considered by some to be an extreme example of a 'performativity' culture, in which particular characteristics of individuals are overemphasized (Evans, Rich, Allwood & Davies, 2007). For example, it could result in characteristics such as physical appearance, performance, competitiveness and victory being viewed as more important than enjoyment, learning, health and social inclusion.

In contexts influenced by performativity culture, young people's body shape, fitness and performance are constantly on display and being evaluated and judged by teachers and peers. Some young people naturally perform well in these evaluations and get rewards (e.g., success, recognition, enjoyment, fun, respect), whereas others perform poorly and receive the sanctions that accompany failure (e.g., discomfort, embarrassment, rejection, harassment, devaluation). Placing emphasis on body shape, weight and size can encourage individuals classified as overweight or obese to be perceived and to perceive themselves as failures, and this process may adversely affect their mental health. With such concerns in mind, some educators argue that it is better to focus on process, or health behaviour, than on product, or health outcome. For example, focusing on being active (or on eating healthily) may be more effective in bringing about behaviour change than focusing on fitness (or weight).

In addition, categorising children as overweight or obese is a complex process, especially as their bodies are growing and maturing. In particular, BMI classifications are not without issues, especially when used with children. At best, BMI provides a general indicator of body fatness, but it is neither reliably accurate nor precise, and it does not predict future body shape and size.

Concerns have also arisen about how information related to children's health (e.g., BMI) is reported to parents and about the expectation for parents to respond to this information. A study exploring the benefits and harms of providing weight feedback to parents as part of the National Child Measurement Programme in England found that providing weight feedback did not cause obvious unfavourable effects and did increase recognition of child overweight and encourage some parents to seek help. However, the effect of weight feedback on behaviour change was limited, which suggested that further work is needed in order to find ways to more effectively communicate health information to parents and identify what information and support might encourage parents to make and maintain lifestyle changes for their children (Falconer et al., 2014).

Alternative Approaches to Monitoring Health in Schools

In addition to conventional ways of monitoring children's health in schools (e.g., measuring height and weight), a range of digital apps are now available that record measurements and provide information and advice about health (including physical activity). Indeed, more than 100,000 health and medical apps are now available through the Apple App Store and Google Play (Lupton, 2014), and they are providing public health knowledge to a range of users. Some of these apps could have merit for use with pupils; however, little is known about how people engage with them, and few of them have been subjected to critical analysis (Lupton, 2014). For this reason, if you wish to employ an app, or indeed any online resource, then you must first evaluate its suitability and utility for young people in terms of its age appropriateness, the health information it provides and the messages it delivers. Some digital resources may be of questionable quality and could confuse or misguide pupils or even promote unhealthy or extreme behaviours. Therefore, you must be a critical and discerning user of such resources and encourage pupils to do likewise.

Learning Through Monitoring Children's Health

Within the curriculum, children learn about their own health and how it is affected by their lifestyle choices. For example, most national curricula require children to learn what they can do to become and stay healthy. They also learn to identify risks and think about their options—and the short- and long-term consequences—when making decisions about personal health. Helping children become aware of, and reflect on, their lifestyle helps them personalise the issue of health and thus makes it meaningful and relevant.

This outcome can be achieved through the use of health behaviour questionnaires, such as those presented in the web resource for this chapter. Responses to such questionnaires can be rated and used to calculate health scores. Here is one possible rating system:

Score 5 points for each 'always' response.

Score 3 points for each 'mostly' response.

Score 2 points for each 'sometimes' response.

Score 0 points for each 'never' response.

Based on their health score total, children can be offered generic feedback such as the following.

- More than 30 points: Congratulations, you lead a very healthy lifestyle and will reap the benefits of doing so, now and in the future. Keep up the good work and try to influence your family and friends to lead a healthy lifestyle too!

- 21 through 30 points: Well done, you lead a healthy lifestyle much of the time and will benefit from doing so. You might consider whether you could lead an even healthier lifestyle by adjusting some of your habits.

- 11 through 20 points: You lead a healthy lifestyle some of the time and will benefit from doing so. However, you should consider leading a healthier lifestyle by improving on a number of your habits.

- 10 or fewer points: Oh dear, it seems that you lead an unhealthy lifestyle and are likely to suffer the consequences, now and in the future. You should consider choosing a much healthier lifestyle by improving on many of your habits.

Applying What You Learn From Monitoring Health

Engaging children in the process of self-reflection enhances learning and helps children to set measurable targets for improvement. Here are some self-reflection questions you might ask of primary-age children:

- Which parts of your health have you done well on?

- Which parts of your health could you do better on?

- Which parts of your health could you change for the better?

- State one action that you can do to improve your health.

And here are some questions for secondary-age children:

- What does your overall health score tell you?

- What have you done well on?

- What could you improve on?

- Are there parts of your health that you cannot change? If yes, what are they?

- What is stopping you from changing these parts?

- What *are* you able to change about your health?

How Healthy Are You? (Secondary Ages)

Health behaviour	Always	Mostly	Sometimes	Never
Do you eat a balanced diet that is low in sugar and fat?				
Do you eat a total of five portions of vegetables and fruits per day?				
Do you drink about six glasses of water per day?				
Do you get enough sleep (about 8 to 10 hours per night)?				
Do you maintain a sensible balance between rest, work and play?				
Are you a nonsmoker?				
Do you drink alcohol in moderation (or not at all)?				
Do you usually remain in control of your emotions?				
Can you adequately cope with the day-to-day pressures and stresses of your work life and personal life?				
Are you active for about an hour every day?				

- State three actions that you can carry out over the next three months to improve your health.
- What will help you carry out these actions?
- What might prevent you from carrying them out?
- On a scale of 0 to 10, how confident are you that you will be able to improve your health over the next three months?

Summary

It is prudent to monitor children's health in schools, both because health-related behaviour patterns are often established during childhood and because schools can influence children's health choices. In one form of monitoring, some countries have established school-based child measurement programmes to address health issues such as obesity. However, these programmes are controversial due to the complexity of categorising children as overweight or obese, the risk of overemphasising individuals' physical characteristics (which can adversely affect their mental health), questions about how information is reported to parents, and issues related to expectations for parents to respond appropriately.

Within the curriculum, children learn about their own health and about the effects of lifestyle choices on their health. Children can be helped to understand what it means to follow a healthy lifestyle by using descriptors of healthy behaviours based on public health recommendations. Children's awareness and understanding of health-related matters can be further enhanced by engaging them in the process of reflecting on their lifestyle. This process can also help them set measurable, manageable targets for improvement.

Monitoring Physical Activity in Schools

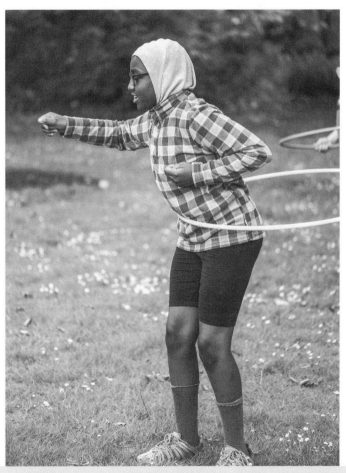

Chapter Objectives

After reading this chapter, you will be able to

- ▶ explain the rationale for monitoring children's physical activity,
- ▶ describe the main methods used for monitoring children's physical activity and their key strengths and limitations,
- ▶ identify ways to promote learning through monitoring children's physical activity and
- ▶ apply practical ideas and tools for monitoring children's physical activity.

While a good deal of attention is paid to monitoring children's physical fitness in school, relatively little attention is given to monitoring their physical *activity*. This chapter addresses that oversight, which constitutes a missed opportunity. First, the chapter considers the rationale for monitoring physical activity and the main methods considered feasible for doing so. It then presents ideas for implementing physical activity monitoring and using it to promote learning and healthy active lifestyles among pupils. This approach enables you to appreciate the value of monitoring pupils' physical activity and equips you with the knowledge, understanding and ideas you need in order to carry it out within your curriculum.

Defining Physical Activity

Physical activity is a broad term defined as any bodily movement produced by skeletal muscles that results in energy expenditure above that required for resting (Trost, 2007). It is important to recognise the difference between physical activity, or body movement, and energy expenditure, which results *from* body movement. Thus, a smaller child and a larger child may engage in the same physical activity (e.g., walking up stairs) but expend a different amount of energy in doing so.

Physical activity encompasses many dimensions and domains. Its dimensions include volume (how much), duration (how long), frequency (how often), intensity (how hard) and mode (what type). Its domains typically include leisure-time physical activity, occupational physical activity, transportation and routine activities performed in and around the house. For children, the domains include physical activity at school and out of school, active travel (e.g., walking, cycling), PE, sport, active play and other activities (e.g., housework, gardening).

Rationale for Monitoring Children's Physical Activity

Monitoring children's physical activity gains importance in light of growing concerns over the physical activity levels of many young people and the strengthening links between physical activity and health reported in chapter 1. More specifi-

cally, it is important to researchers and clinicians for the following reasons (Trost, 2007; Loprinzi & Cardinal, 2011):

- To establish the physical activity patterns of various population groups
- To understand the links between physical activity and health
- To establish the amount of physical activity required to influence overall health and specific health outcomes
- To identify and understand the factors that influence physical activity
- To evaluate the effectiveness of interventions related to physical activity

A number of purposes have also been identified for monitoring children's physical activity in schools (Cale & Harris, 2009), including:

- To determine how active pupils are and whether they are meeting current physical activity recommendations (as discussed in chapter 1)
- To raise children's awareness and understanding of their own (and recommended) levels of physical activity and thus assist with target setting and behaviour change
- To help meet curriculum aims and requirements related to being physically active and leading healthy, active lives through enhanced awareness and understanding
- To determine the effect of physical activity initiatives and strategies implemented by schools
- To contribute to a broader and more holistic approach to monitoring, which goes beyond clinical and fitness outcomes by also considering behaviours and physical activity as a process (For more on the limitations of focusing only on physical fitness, see chapter 6.)

Methods of Monitoring Children's Physical Activity

Numerous methods can be used to monitor children's physical activity with varying levels of sophistication and various strengths and limitations. Over the years, a number of comprehensive method reviews have been published (e.g., Dollman et al., 2009; Kohl, Fulton, & Caspersen, 2000; Trost, 2007; Loprinzi & Cardinal, 2011). This discussion outlines the methods considered to be most practical and effective for use with pupils. These methods can be grouped broadly as follows:

- Self-reports and proxy reports
- Heart rate monitoring
- Pedometers and accelerometers
- Observation

Self-Reports and Proxy Reports

Self-report probably remains the most commonly used method of monitoring children's physical activity. Self-report measures that are well suited for use with children include surveys and questionnaires (which can be self- or interviewer-administered), diaries and proxy reports (in which parents or teachers report on children's activity).

Self-report measures vary greatly in the nature of physical activity information they collect (e.g., type, duration, intensity, frequency), the timescale covered (e.g., one year, one week, one day) and how the results are reported (e.g., activity score, minutes in activity). Self-report measures typically offer the following main strengths:

- Convenient and easy to administer
- Time- and cost-efficient
- Suitable for providing information about type and context of physical activity
- Not burdensome
- Unobtrusive and nonreactive (thus unlikely to alter observed behaviour)

At the same time, self-report measures are subject to some limitations relating to, for example, the respondent's (particularly, child's) recall ability, interpretation and honesty, as well as varying levels of appropriateness for capturing certain types of activity (e.g., unstructured play).

Despite these limitations, evidence suggests that self-report methods provide acceptable estimates of physical activity in older children. They are less accurate and less reliable, however, with children under the age of 10. For primary-age children, more appropriate approaches include proxy reports and objective measures, such as accelerometers (Trost, 2007; Loprinzi & Cardinal, 2011).

Various self-report measures have been developed for use with children, and they have been summarised and evaluated for reliability and validity in a number of reviews (e.g., Sallis & Saelens, 2000; Kohl et al., 2000; Biddle, Gorely, Pearson, & Bull, 2011). Self-report instruments that have been identified and endorsed in the literature include the Previous Day Physical Activity Recall (PDPAR), the Three-Day Physical Activity Recall (3DPAR), the Physical Activity Questionnaire for Children (PAQ-C) or for Adolescents (PAQ-A), the Youth Risk Behavior Surveillance System (YRBSS) and the Teen Health Survey (for more information about these instruments, see Trost [2007] and Biddle et al. [2011]). A caveat: It has been suggested that the large number of self-report instruments highlighted in reviews illustrates a lack of uniformity in approach and suggests that investigators feel compelled to design their own instruments (Trost, 2007).

Heart Rate Monitoring

Another commonly used method for estimating children's physical activity is heart rate monitoring. It is considered a feasible and attractive method because it relies on the strong relationship between heart rate and energy expenditure during exercise. Modern heart rate monitors usually comprise two elements: a chest strap transmitter and a wrist receiver (which usually doubles as a watch) or mobile phone. Many systems and designs are now commercially available, and they provide various types of information—for example, average heart rate; breathing rate; time spent in, at or above a specific heart rate; and detailed logging that can be downloaded to a computer.

Heart rate monitoring offers a number of advantages, such as the following:

- The monitors are small, relatively cheap, robust, easy to use and socially acceptable.
- The method is unobtrusive, does not restrict movement and should not influence normal activity.
- Information can be collected for long periods of time.
- It provides physiological quantification of physical activity in a manner that is both valid and reliable.

Drawbacks of heart rate monitoring include the following:

- It does not provide a direct measure of physical activity but represents the individual's physiological response to activity.
- Heart rate is influenced by many factors, such as age, body size, fitness level, metabolism, emotional state, fatigue, temperature, type of exercise and muscle mass used.
- The relationship between heart rate and energy expenditure is weak during low- or high-intensity physical activity.
- Heart rate response lags behind changes in movement and may therefore mask the intermittent activity of children.
- The method may be of limited use for assessing children's total daily physical activity when most of their day is spent being inactive.

Pedometers and Accelerometers

Pedometers provide an estimate of overall physical activity and are well suited to measuring children's physical activity. They are generally worn on the hip or waist and rely on the vertical movements of the body to count the number of steps taken over a period of time. A variety of models are available that have been found to provide valid and reliable assessments of children's physical activity.

Key advantages of pedometers include the fact that they are

- small, easy to use and socially acceptable;
- cost effective and
- unobtrusive and thus do not restrict movement or influence normal activity.

Disadvantages of pedometers include the fact that they

- provide limited activity information (e.g., provide no information about activity type, pattern or intensity);
- are not suitable for monitoring some types of activities—for example, ones that do not involve travel or impact (e.g., cycling, rowing, throwing and catching) and
- count movement above a certain threshold as a step regardless of whether or not it occurs during walking or running.

Accelerometers are more sophisticated than pedometers and are considered to be the most promising objective tools for measuring physical activity in free-living children (Trost, 2007). Usually worn on the hip, these devices record the vertical accelerations of the body produced by movement at specific time intervals and convert them to an activity count. In general, accelerometers share many of the same advantages and disadvantages as pedometers, but they offer the added advantage of being able to assess the frequency, duration and intensity of movement. A number of accelerometers are now available, and they vary in both sophistication and cost.

Technological advances in the consumer health and fitness market have also led to a proliferation of other wearable electronic devices (e.g., Fitbit). They generally consist of an accelerometer for measuring physical activity, as well as secondary sensors that provide additional information and feedback on various aspects of activity.

Observation

Observation enables direct measurement of physical activity and is particularly well suited to monitoring children's physical activity in the school context. It usually involves watching a child for an extended period of time and recording a rating of the child's activity level on either a coding form or a handheld device. Activity category ratings are usually recorded at time intervals ranging from every five seconds to every minute. Various systems for direct observation have been developed over the years for use in school and physical education lessons, as well as general settings. Two widely used tools are the System for Observing Play and Leisure Activity in Youth (SOPLAY) and the Observational System for Recording Physical Activity in Children (OSRAC). For details of these and other systems, see Trost (2007) and Kohl et al. (2000).

Observation offers the following major advantages:

- It can provide accurate, detailed information that covers type, intensity and duration of physical activity and the physical and social context of activity, such as behavioural cues, environmental conditions and the presence of significant others or of toys and equipment.
- It is flexible and can be used in a variety of settings.

- It is particularly appropriate for young children's activity, which is often sporadic and transitory.
- Observers can be easily trained to record accurate information.

Disadvantages of observation include the following:

- The activity recorded is limited to what is seen; therefore, significant information may be missed.
- There are limits to where and when activity can be observed.
- The potential exists for reactivity among the children; that is, they may alter their behaviour due to being observed.
- Observation is burdensome and time- and labour-intensive.

Thus, you can choose from a number of measures when looking to monitor physical activity levels. As just outlined, all of the methods have both strengths and limitations, and no single method can be considered optimal in all situations. Therefore, we will always be faced with a trade-off between practicality and accuracy when selecting a monitoring tool to use with young people (Trost, 2007). Research, of course, requires an accurate measure of physical activity. As a result, given that all methods are subject to limitations, it has been recommended that researchers use a combination of methods in order to provide a more accurate and complete picture of children's activity levels. However, when teachers are choosing a measure of physical activity for use with pupils, the accuracy that researchers try to achieve is not required; instead, issues such as educational value, cost, feasibility and ease of use are more important.

To inform decisions about which methods to use, Trost (2007) has provided a useful summary of monitoring methods that addresses key attributes such as validity, affordability, ease of administration, potential for reactivity, and feasibility with large numbers and various ages. In addition, Dollman et al. (2009) have developed a decision flow chart to help both researchers and practitioners select appropriate monitoring methods. When monitoring physical activity in schools as part of the curriculum, educational value is more important than some other attributes, and the limitations of a measure should not be seen as devaluing the assessment. Rather than worrying unduly about the precision of the method, it is more important pedagogically to ensure that pupils learn from the experience (Cale & Harris, 2009).

Learning Through Monitoring Children's Physical Activity

Having identified measures that are considered feasible and practical for use with pupils, we can now consider some ideas for incorporating these measures within the curriculum. As noted in chapter 4, children learn about health and healthy lifestyles within the curriculum, and this learning includes physical activity and active lifestyles. As with their lifestyles in general, increasing children's awareness of their physical activity levels makes the notion of healthy active lifestyles meaningful and relevant. This goal can be achieved through any of the following methods, which have been adapted and developed from preexisting ideas (Cale & Harris, 2009).

Self-Report

The self-report questionnaire is often the easiest method of physical activity monitoring to incorporate into lessons. As appropriate, you can use or adapt an existing questionnaire on paper (e.g., PDPAR, 3DPAR, PAQ-C or PAQ-A, Teen Health Survey). Many researchers, however, design their own questionnaires, and this option is also feasible for teachers and allows them to tailor the form and questions to their specific school context, pupils and needs. Pupils can even be asked to develop their own physical activity questionnaires, which requires them to understand what type of information is useful to establish.

You can get a quick, simple indication of pupils' physical activity levels by asking general questions about their physical activity (Cale & Harris, 2009). Here is an example:

During a one-week period, how many times on average do you do the following kind of physical activity?

Vigorous activity: Involves lots of effort and makes your heart beat fast—for example, basketball, football, jogging, running, energetic dancing, aerobics or circuit training.

Moderate activity: Makes you warm and slightly out of breath but not exhausted—for example, brisk walking, steady swimming, cycling or dancing.

Light activity: Involves little effort—for example, walking, bowling or snooker.

(Cale & Harris, 2009, p. 92)

Another approach would be to ask pupils whether they do any of the specific physical activities included in a predetermined list—and if so, how often. The list should include a range of activities suitable to the pupils' age that can be done both in and outside of school; it can even be devised with pupils' input. Options for indicating how often the activities are done might include: not at all, once a week, a few times a week, every day or more. For primary-age children, the list of activities might include any or all of the following: walking, cycling, skipping, tag, chase, ball games, swimming, dance and football. For secondary-age children, the activities might include walking, cycling, jogging, running, aerobics, circuits, yoga, martial arts, swimming, dance, football, hockey, rugby, basketball, badminton, tennis and skateboarding or other street activities. To capture any unlisted activities that pupils do, you can provide an 'Other Activities' line for them to fill in.

Another idea is to ask pupils to keep a daily physical activity diary for a specified period of time, such as a week, a month or a unit of work. The minimum information to record in the diary each day would typically include the number, types and duration (in minutes) of physical activities engaged in. Upper-primary or secondary children might also be asked to record the intensity of their activities (e.g., low or light, average or moderate, or vigorous or hard), as well as where the activities were performed and with whom. This information can be recorded in either a free diary format or a more structured one, examples of which can be seen in the web resource for this chapter.

Pupils can also be encouraged to write a short narrative, profile or blog about their own physical activity levels and patterns (and possibly their experiences of particular activities). These accounts are likely to generate a range of physical activity profiles that can be used to prompt discussion.

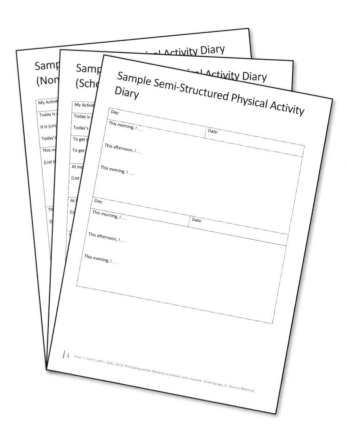

Heart Rate Monitoring

Heart rate monitors are now quite affordable and have been used frequently in physical education, notably to help pupils learn about how exercise affects the body and about target heart rate ranges. Of course, they can also be used to monitor pupils' heart rates, and therefore their activity levels, either during lessons, over the course of a school day or for a more extended period (e.g., a school week). Depending on how many devices are available for a given class, this approach might be used for a selection of pupils at any given time; then, with those pupils' permission, the data could be shared and discussed with the whole class.

Pedometers and Accelerometers

Pedometers and accelerometers can now be purchased easily and at relatively low cost, and they can be used with pupils in much the same way as heart rate monitors. Some electronic devices (e.g., Fitbit) also provide additional information and feedback with which pupils can readily engage. These devices, which consist of an accelerometer that works with a digital app, go beyond measuring and self-monitoring physical activity to provide information, feedback and advice and to facilitate goal setting. Indeed, one review of available options for self-monitoring identified more than 80 such devices that can be used by researchers, clinicians and members of the general public (Sanders et al., 2016). If you wish to employ such devices with pupils, consider both their utility and their suitability (in terms of age appropriateness, activity information provided and messages advocated) and encourage pupils to be discerning consumers and users of these tools.

Observation

Valuable information about physical activity can be obtained through direct observation without adopting a complicated system. Simple observation forms can be prepared for recording and coding the details of activity, including type, intensity and duration. Pupils can be paired up and asked to observe and record the partner's physical activity during a school day or week by tracking his or her movements during lessons, breaks and lunchtimes and after school. The information can then be shared and discussed as a small- or whole-group activity.

Further advances in learning through monitoring include an increased focus on children's sedentary behaviour. This focus is advocated for a few reasons:

- increases in the amount of time that children spend engaged in sedentary behaviour (Salmon, Tremblay, Marshall, & Hume, 2011),
- growing evidence of links between sedentary behaviour and health (Wilmot et al., 2012) and
- recent physical activity guidelines focus on reducing sedentary time (see chapter 1).

Sedentary behaviour is often assessed by noting the amount of time that children spend

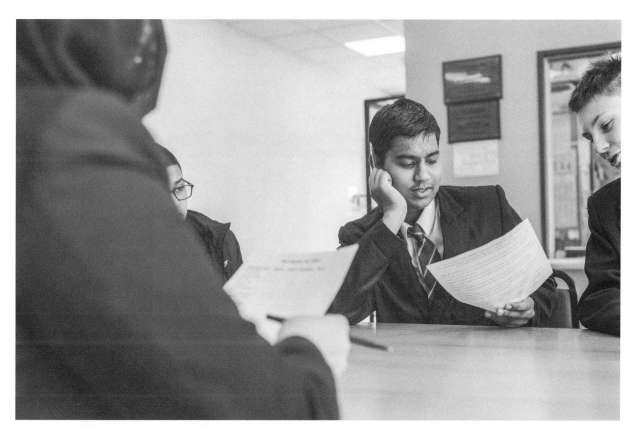

Teachers can guide pupils to reflect on their activity levels and to set targets to help adopt active lifestyles.

watching television or engaged in other screen-based activities, such as using a computer or playing video games (Loprinzi & Cardinal, 2011). Various methods have been used to measure screen-based behaviour, including self- and proxy reports, questionnaires, diaries and observation. Whilst screen time provides only a partial picture of overall sedentary time—excluding, for example, non-computer-based homework and socialising—you can usefully incorporate screen-time reports into existing physical measures. The information gathered about pupils' sedentary behaviour can also be used to promote discussion about inactivity and activity.

In summary, you can be as creative as you wish both in how you monitor pupils' physical activity (and sedentary) behaviour and in how you use the resulting information. See the following case study for one school's approach to monitoring physical activity, as well as some sample discussion points.

Applying What You Learn From Monitoring Physical Activity

Once you have obtained physical activity information, it can be used to prompt discussion, reflection and further questions about physical activity in general and about pupils' activities

PHYSICAL ACTIVITY PASSPORT

One school in the East Midlands introduced an incentive scheme known as the Physical Activity Passport as a way to both monitor and promote pupils' physical activity during a summer term. All pupils were given a passport, in which they collected stamps over a given period of time by participating in physical activities, sport clubs, matches and events at school. The stamps (coloured stickers) were distributed by teachers present at the various activities. Pupils also used their passport pages to record any other physical activities in which they took part, whether in or outside of school, and whether structured or unstructured. Upon collecting a set numbers of stamps, pupils were rewarded for their participation with small to medium-size gifts, such as a pen, a water bottle, a baseball cap, a piece of play or sport equipment (e.g., ball, flying disc, skipping rope) or a leisure centre voucher. The passports were also used to prompt discussion during physical education lessons; during tutor time with the class teacher; and during personal, social, health and economic education lessons.

Discussion points: What are your views on the range of gifts offered? Could a focus on extrinsic rewards such as gifts diminish the intrinsic value of physical activity?

At the end of the summer term, the school evaluated the scheme's effects from the perspectives of both pupils and teachers. With regards to pupils, more than 90 percent engaged with the scheme and collected some stamps in their passports, and 75 percent gathered enough stamps for a small reward. In addition, more than 60 percent reported that the scheme had encouraged them and their friends to do more activity and made them more aware of which sports, clubs and activities were available to them, both in and out of school. Furthermore, more than 90 percent of pupils said they felt that the scheme was a good idea, and most indicated that they had enjoyed it and thought it should be run again. Responses from the teachers were also positive; specifically, the majority felt that it should continue and reported it to be relatively easy to implement, as well as fun and enjoyable.

Given the scheme's initial success, the school is planning to run and possibly further develop the scheme for next year. For example, teachers are considering introducing a Class Passport Challenge, wherein the aim will be for classes or year groups to collect as many stamps as possible. Those with the most stamps will be rewarded with a trip to a sporting event or other activity of their choice, such as bowling, ice skating, karting, paintballing or a visit to an aqua or leisure park. Another possible development is to introduce a Family Passport Challenge to encourage involvement by parents and other family members.

Discussion points: What might be the pros and cons of incorporating the Class Passport Challenge or a Family Passport Challenge? What other developments or improvements might be used to enhance the scheme?

and lifestyles in particular. Of course, the amount and depth of coverage will need to vary and be adapted according to the pupils' ages and abilities. Here are some ways to use such information to facilitate pupils' learning:

- To enhance pupils' knowledge and understanding of physical activity—for example, the importance of physical activity, what it means to be physically active, how much and what types of physical activity are recommended for health, how physical activity is affected by factors both within and beyond an individual's control, key constraints and barriers to participation and how they can be overcome, and what can be achieved collectively and individually to improve physical activity levels nationwide

- To develop pupils' personal physical activity awareness and knowledge—for example, about their current activity levels and patterns, sedentary behaviour, interests and preferences—and their self-evaluation skills, so that they can understand, interpret, plan and make informed decisions about their physical activity (Sample questions to ask pupils are outlined in the web resource under the heading Thinking About Your Physical Activity.)

- To facilitate pupils' goal setting and self-monitoring of physical activity—for example, using the information as the basis for setting realistic goals to increase or maintain their physical activity levels, reduce their sedentary behaviour and work towards meeting physical activity recommendations for young people (See chapter 1 and the Thinking About Your Physical Activity questions in the web resource for this chapter.)

- To diagnose pupils' activity needs for individual exercise prescription based on their current physical activity levels and the extent to which they are meeting current physical activity recommendations

- To help pupils develop broader and more transferable skills (e.g., independent inquiry, critical reflection, problem solving, self-management) and cross-curricular skills and links between subjects (e.g., physical education, science, literacy, numeracy, statistics)

The information gained from activity monitoring will enhance your understanding of your pupils' physical activity levels, patterns, interests

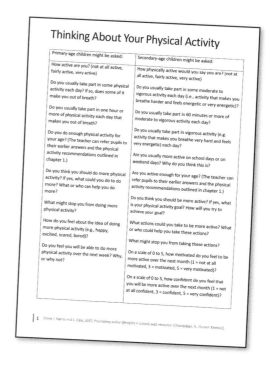

and preferences. You can use this understanding to inform the curriculum and the range of curricular and extracurricular activities you offer; the types of initiatives and programmes you choose to run in your particular school; and the community links you choose to continue or develop with local leisure centres and sport (or other appropriate) clubs and organisations.

Summary

It is important to monitor children's physical activity both because of its health benefits and because of concerns about low levels of participation in activity. Monitoring children's physical activity in schools raises pupils' awareness and understanding of their own levels and of recommended levels of physical activity; it also helps with target setting and behaviour change. Numerous monitoring methods exist—including self- and proxy reports, heart rate monitoring, use of pedometers or accelerometers, and observation. Because each method has its own strengths and limitations, no single method is optimal for all situations. Information can also be gathered through the use of health and physical activity apps and computer-based physical activity questionnaires, providing that you carefully consider their suitability and appropriateness for your pupils. Monitoring efforts have expanded recently to include children's *sedentary* behaviours via self- and proxy reports, questionnaires, diaries and observation.

When choosing methods for monitoring, factors to consider include educational value, cost, and feasibility. Monitoring physical activity can facilitate pupils' learning by developing their physical activity awareness and knowledge and their self-evaluation skills. It can also facilitate goal setting and self-monitoring of physical activity.

Monitoring Physical Fitness in Schools

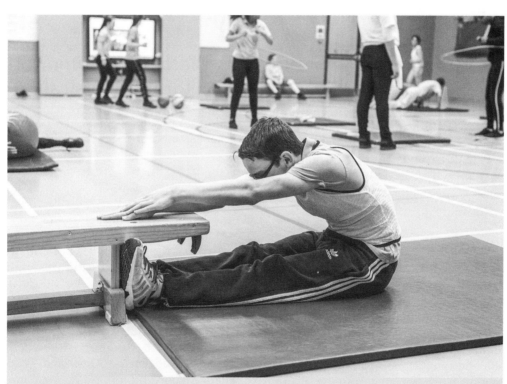

Chapter Objectives

After reading this chapter, you will be able to

- explain the rationale proposed for monitoring children's physical fitness,
- describe methods of monitoring children's physical fitness that are appropriate for use in schools and in the curriculum,
- identify ways to promote learning through monitoring children's physical fitness,
- understand common issues and concerns associated with monitoring children's physical fitness and
- apply recommendations and practical ideas for the appropriate use of fitness monitoring.

Monitoring children's physical fitness in schools is commonplace in secondary schools and is even mandatory in some countries. However, its purpose, value and place in the curriculum remain topics of much debate. To help you understand this debate, this chapter examines controversial issues associated with fitness testing in schools. The chapter also presents recommendations and practical ideas to help you make informed decisions about fitness monitoring and employ effective and appropriate monitoring practices.

Defining Physical Fitness

Physical fitness has been defined as a set of attributes involving the ability to perform physical activity; it is often described in terms of either health-related or performance-related (skill-related) components (Caspersen, Powell, & Christenson, 1985). Health-related components of physical fitness are associated with specific health outcomes (Pate, 1988) and comprise cardiorespiratory fitness, muscular strength and endurance, flexibility and body composition.

Rationale for Monitoring Children's Physical Fitness

Many reasons for monitoring children's physical fitness have been put forward over the years. For example, researchers collect fitness data in order to better understand children's fitness levels, fitness phenomena and their demography; to establish baseline measures for analysing the health-related fitness of a group or population; and to investigate the effects of training on children's fitness. In the clinical setting, fitness monitoring allows practitioners to evaluate medical abnormalities, assess symptoms associated with exercise, measure exercise capacity and individualise physical activity programmes (Cale & Harris, 2005). Indeed, the growing link between health-related fitness and health outcomes in children (Lloyd, Colley, & Tremblay, 2010) has strengthened the rationale for monitoring children's physical fitness and indicates potential value in promoting and monitoring not only children's physical activity but also their physical fitness.

In schools, fitness testing can potentially serve a number of purposes, including the following:

- Promoting physical activity
- Developing skills in goal setting, self-monitoring and self-testing
- Promoting learning and positive attitudes
- Motivating pupils
- Evaluating fitness programmes
- Identifying pupils with athletic potential
- Screening pupils for health issues
- Diagnosing fitness needs for individual exercise prescription and improvement

(Cale & Harris, 2009b, p. 59).

Methods of Monitoring Children's Physical Fitness

Children's physical fitness can be monitored in either the laboratory or the field; either way, the monitoring is usually conducted through a range of standard fitness tests. In the field, fitness testing typically involves administering a battery of simple tests that cover various components of fitness, and this approach is the most practical option for monitoring in schools.

Physical fitness includes both **health-related components** and **performance-related (skill-related) components**. As the term implies, health-related components relate to health outcomes, and they include **cardiorespiratory fitness**, **muscular strength and endurance**, **flexibility** and **body composition**. Performance-related aspects, on the other hand, include agility, balance, coordination, power, reaction time and speed; this type of fitness is sometimes referred to as **motor fitness**. Some evidence suggests that performance-related components also relate to health; however, because they are influenced by physical ability, we focus here on health-related components assessed via field-based tests. The following discussion covers some of the most popular tests for each component of health-related fitness (for a quick summary, see table 6.1).

Cardiorespiratory Fitness

Distance runs have been commonly used as a field measure of cardiorespiratory fitness in children.

TABLE 6.1 Common Field Tests of Physical Fitness for Children

Fitness component	Field tests
Cardiorespiratory fitness	Distance or timed walk or run (e.g., 1 mile, 1.5 miles; 9 minutes, 12 minutes)
	Step test
	Multistage fitness test
Muscular strength and endurance	Sit-ups or curl-ups (abdominals)
	Progressive abdominal sit-up (curl) test
	Push-ups or press-ups (triceps, pectorals)
	Pull-ups (biceps)
	Flexed-arm hang (biceps)
Flexibility	Sit-and-reach (hip)
	Shoulder stretch (shoulder)
	Arm lift (shoulder)
Body composition	Body mass index (BMI)
	Skinfold thickness
	Girth measures

Examples include the mile run or walk (in which children complete the distance as quickly as possible) and the 9- or 12-minute distance run (in which children run as far as they can in the given time). Another common method, the multistage fitness or 'bleep' test, is a progressive shuttle run that predicts maximum oxygen uptake. Because it requires the individual to run to exhaustion (and for other reasons outlined later in the chapter), this test has been the subject of questions about its appropriateness for use with children, particularly its use with all pupils and within curriculum time (Association for Physical Education [afPE], 2016; Cale, Harris, & Chen, 2014).

Muscular Strength and Endurance

Field tests of muscular strength and endurance involve resisting or moving part or all of one's body weight. The areas of the body most often tested for strength and endurance include the stomach (abdominals) and the upper arms and chest (triceps, biceps and pectorals). They are tested through exercises such as sit-ups, curl-ups, push-ups, press-ups, pull-ups and the flexed-arm hang. These tests usually involve performing as many repetitions as possible in a given time or before the muscles involved reach their limit. One example of the latter approach is the progressive abdominal sit-up test, in which the individual per-

forms curl-ups to a controlled and timed 'bleep' until unable to continue. Thus, like the progressive shuttle run, it is a maximal test; therefore, questions can be raised about its appropriateness for use with all children within curriculum time.

Flexibility

The most common field measure of flexibility involves assessing the range of motion at the hip joint by means of the sit-and-reach test. This test is common because poor flexibility in the lower back and hamstring region can cause low-back pain. Other common flexibility tests include the shoulder stretch and the arm lift, which assess range of motion at the shoulder joint.

Body Composition

In the field, body composition is typically estimated by using anthropometry, or measurement of the body's dimensions. One commonly used measure is **body mass index** (BMI), which is derived from the individual's weight (body mass) and height. Another common measure is skinfold thickness, which indicates body fatness. In children, skinfold measurements are usually taken from a few selected areas of the body—often the triceps (back of the upper arm), biceps (front of the upper arm), subscapular (beneath the edge

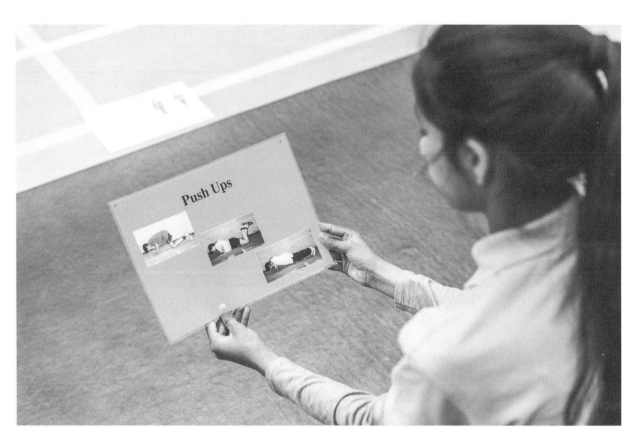

Teachers can guide pupils to reflect on their fitness levels and to set targets to help adopt active lifestyles.

of the shoulder blade), suprailiac (just above the hip bone), front thigh and medial calf. The sum of the skinfold measurements is then used as an indication of total body fat. When monitoring children's body composition, it is important to be aware of the sensitivities and potential issues of doing so (these concerns are addressed later in the chapter).

Learning Through Monitoring Children's Physical Fitness

The educational worth of fitness monitoring can be considered in terms of what young people learn, both from the experience and from the resulting information, as well as the effects on their physical activity, fitness and attitudes (Cale, 2016). At the same time, as noted earlier, fitness monitoring of children has generated debate about a number of issues and concerns. Therefore, before considering how fitness monitoring might be used to promote learning, let us consider a brief critique of fitness testing in terms of the advantages, disadvantages, issues and cautions.

This critique will help inform your decisions and practices with respect to fitness monitoring and, in turn, your pupils' experiences of and learning through monitoring.

When looking to monitor pupils' fitness, we must bear in mind a number of advantages and disadvantages that are common to all fitness tests and test batteries. Key advantages include the following:

- The tests are generally easy to administer and time efficient.
- The tests are relatively safe and involve minimal equipment and cost.
- Scientific evidence supports many of the tests and their use with children.
- Much testing now emphasises the evaluation of health-related components.
- Tests can provide useful information about children's capabilities in a range of fitness components.
- Many tests are supported by educational programmes and attractive resources, materials and software.

(Cale & Harris, 2009b).

And here are some key disadvantages:

- Field tests provide a relatively crude measure of an individual's physical fitness.
- Reliability and validity are questionable in some tests for use with children.
- Fitness test batteries with children frequently use **norm-referenced standards** and **criterion-referenced standards**, which are subject to some limitations (this topic is addressed later in the chapter).
- Children's performance on fitness tests is influenced by many factors, such as environmental conditions (e.g., temperature, humidity, wind speed and direction), test procedures, lifestyle (exercise and nutrition), motivation, intellectual and physical skill in test taking, heredity (genetic potential) and level of maturation (Cale & Harris, 2009b, pp. 61–62).

The influence exerted by each of these factors varies, both between tests and between monitoring sessions. Generally, however, heredity (genetic potential) and maturation are reported to exert the most influence on fitness test results (Cale & Harris, 2009b).

Concerns About Fitness Monitoring

As noted by Cale and Harris (2009b, p. 62), it has been claimed that 'fitness tests simply determine the obvious, at best only distinguishing the mature and/or motivated from the immature and/or unmotivated' and 'between those "blessed" with "fit" genes at birth and those not so blessed'. Although such disadvantages are not necessarily problematic in themselves, they are clearly relevant when promoting learning through fitness monitoring—specifically, when interpreting results and deciding what information, key messages and feedback to provide to pupils along with the test results. In addition, many of the concerns raised about fitness monitoring relate not to the tests or to monitoring per se but to testing practices. In other words, they relate to how monitoring is carried out, the purposes of monitoring and potential negative consequences for pupils.

Mode of Implementation

Concerns have been expressed over the way in which fitness monitoring is often implemented within the curriculum. For example, fitness testing is sometimes treated as an almost irrelevant adjunct to the curriculum. In other cases, it dominates or even constitutes the entire fitness education programme. This imbalance is considered particularly important if fitness testing comes at the expense of promoting the process of being active; providing activity-promoting activities; or developing pupils' knowledge and understanding of physical activity, physical fitness and the monitoring of these elements. This type of imbalance can give the impression that physical fitness is more important than health and physical activity, which in turn can lead to overemphasis on fitness and performance and not enough on health and physical activity behaviour. In contrast, from the point of view of public health and the promotion of physical activity, it has been argued that the goal should be to influence the process of physical activity rather than the product of fitness (Cale & Harris, 2009b). In fact, influencing the process (activity) should exert a positive influence on the product (fitness).

False Assumptions

Concerns have also been raised about some common assumptions underlying fitness and fitness monitoring, the messages these assumptions might generate, and the possible consequences for pupils. First, there is little evidence to support the commonly held view and rationale for fitness monitoring that it promotes healthy lifestyles and physical activity, motivates young people, and develops the knowledge and skills that are important to sustain engagement in an active lifestyle (Cale & Harris, 2009b). To the contrary, researchers have expressed concerns that fitness testing can be counterproductive to achieving this goal. Specifically, it may be unpleasant, uncomfortable, embarrassing and seemingly meaningless for many young people; moreover, scores can be inaccurate, misleading, unfair and demotivating and therefore switch many individuals off of rather than onto activity (Cale & Harris, 2009b; Keating, 2003; Rice, 2007; Naughton, Carlson, & Greene, 2006). This concern led Cale and Harris (2009a) to conclude that fitness testing may well represent a misdirected effort in the promotion of healthy lifestyles and that time could therefore be better spent otherwise.

Another commonly held inaccurate assumption is that fitness in children primarily reflects the amount of physical activity in which they engage and, in turn, that those who do well on fitness tests are active and that those who do poorly are inactive. In reality, the relationship between physical fitness and physical activity is low among children, and a child's activity level cannot be judged from his or her fitness level (Cale & Harris, 2009b). Whilst physical activity can, as noted earlier, make a positive and important contribution to an individual's fitness, physical fitness is also influenced by other factors, such as maturation and genetics (heredity). Indeed, it can be problematic to link pupils' fitness test scores to their activity levels: 'On the one hand, an active student who scores badly on a test may become disappointed, disillusioned, demotivated and switched off activity because he/she feels it does not pay off. Equally, an inactive student who scores well may be delighted with the result, conclude that everything is fine when it is not, and consequently, may not be motivated to change' (Cale & Harris, 2009b, p. 65).

Questionable Fitness Tests and Test Practices

In theory, fitness monitoring can be used to advocate safe and healthy practices, yet some fitness test batteries and practices involve children in performing tests that arguably violate healthy behaviour and, in the view of some observers, common sense (Cale & Harris, 2009b). For example, questionable practices cited in one study included the use of maximal fitness tests (most notably the multistage fitness test), the public posting of fitness test scores (thus allowing pupils to compare performances) and the monitoring of pupils' weight or body composition (Cale, Harris, & Chen, 2014). Concern about using the multistage fitness test with children focuses on the fact that it was developed for use with elite adult populations, carries an element of risk and can be overly public and misused, which in turn can undermine the confidence of, and embarrass, some youngsters (Cale, 2016). Displaying fitness test scores in order to enable comparisons also seems inappropriate given the many factors known to influence fitness test performance and test scores such as environmental conditions, heredity and level of maturation (Cale, Harris, & Chen, 2014).

The third area of concern—the weighing and measuring of children—is clearly a sensitive issue. Overemphasis on this practice could lead to body dissatisfaction, the development of harmful relationships with food, and, in some cases, disordered eating. These are serious and increasing problems in many countries, particularly among adolescents and, more specifically, adolescent girls. On this issue, Cale and Harris (2009b, p.143) have argued that 'it is not necessary to measure any individual to tell them something that they already know, and more importantly, no child needs to be measured to be helped to enjoy being physically active'; moreover, 'overemphasising "fat" measurements may simply contribute a mental health problem to a physical health issue'.

Interpretation and Use of Fitness Monitoring Data

The practice of applying norm-referenced or criterion-referenced standards when interpreting fitness test results is common and has been critiqued in more detail elsewhere (e.g., Cale & Harris, 2005, 2009b). Normative standards involve comparing a child's score with that of a reference group, whereas criterion-referenced standards are absolute and specify the minimum levels of fitness thought to be required for health and for performing daily tasks. Criterion-referenced standards are considered most attractive from theoretical, pedagogical and philosophical points of view because they clearly identify the existence of a level of fitness (below that needed to be an elite athlete) that is sufficient to maintain health. They are also informative in broadly categorizing individuals as either working towards, meeting or exceeding minimum standards.

At the same time, the use of criterion-referenced and norm-referenced standards is subject to limitations. For example, the validity of some criterion-referenced standards is questionable or unknown and may seem somewhat arbitrary; this could provide some pupils with little incentive to move towards meeting the stated desirable minimum levels of fitness. Furthermore, the use of arbitrary criterion-referenced standards could lead to misclassification of pupils' fitness levels. Norm tables are also limited in that they do not indicate desired levels of physical fitness or provide diagnostic feedback about whether one's fitness level is adequate; in addition, they imply that 'more is always better'.

As schools face increasing pressure to assess and demonstrate pupil progress across curriculum subjects, including physical education, it seems (anecdotally) more commonplace to see baseline testing and fitness monitoring draw on various norm- and criterion- referenced standards. However, it is considered inappropriate to use fitness monitoring simply to obtain fitness test data or to grade pupils as a primary indicator of their progress and achievement (Cale & Harris, 2009b). Not only does it represent a very narrow measure of achievement and reduce a complex concept to raw figures, which is limiting in itself, but also it is likely to constitute a limiting learning experience with undesirable consequences for pupils. For example, it could lead to a loss of interest in physical education and physical activity; a 'teaching to the test' mentality; cheating; or the undermining of confidence in pupils who find that, even with effort, they fail to achieve good grades or meet expectations due to the various factors beyond their control that influence fitness test scores (Cale & Harris, 2009b). Furthermore, if fitness performances and scores are subject to grading and comparisons, then testing may also give pupils the false message that competition and excellence are necessary for health and fitness. This message alone may deter some from wishing to participate and thus hinder efforts to promote physical activity.

Fitness Monitoring Recommendations

These issues and concerns are not presented to dissuade you from monitoring children's fitness but to highlight the fact that positive outcomes from monitoring (including learning) cannot be taken for granted and that there are pitfalls to be aware of when monitoring. Lloyd et al. (2010) argue that fear of fitness assessment should not be allowed to outweigh the potential benefits of the information obtained and the pedagogical value to pupils. Therefore, rather than being overly critical of fitness monitoring due to its limitations, we should reflect on and promote good pedagogical practice in this regard.

Indeed, the consensus from many sources seems to be that if fitness monitoring is used appropriately, subjected to informed critique that accounts for its limitations, and incorporated as one component of a broad and holistic health education programme, then it can serve as a valuable part of the curriculum and play a role in supporting healthy lifestyles and physical activity (afPE, 2015a; Cale, 2016; Cale & Harris, 2009a; Cale, Harris, & Chen, 2014; Lloyd et al., 2010; Rowland, 2007; Silverman, Keating, & Phillips, 2008). In order to meet these criteria, monitoring should be developmentally appropriate; offer a positive, educational experience for all learners; and help promote healthy, active lifestyles.

In terms of developmental appropriateness, it is questionable whether fitness monitoring and fitness testing are appropriate for primary-age children or for children under the age of nine. In this regard, in response to a recommendation to introduce fitness testing in primary schools, the Association for Physical Education (afPE, 2015b) published a position statement declaring that it does not support formal fitness testing in primary schools; to the contrary, the group considers such testing to be a retrograde step in terms of promoting healthy, active lifestyles.

Ensuring best practice when monitoring fitness requires training, guidance, support and opportunities for open and supportive professional dialogue (Cale, 2016), elements of which are provided in this chapter. In addition, recommendations and guidelines for fitness testing with young people have been published by various authors and organisations over the years. Examples include the American College of Sports Medicine; the American Alliance for Health, Physical Education, Recreation and Dance (now SHAPE America: the Society of Health and Physical Educators); the Association for Physical Education; Silverman et al. (2008); Cale & Harris (2009b); and Cale, Harris, & Chen (2014).

More recent recommendations have been informed by, adapted, or developed from previous ones (e.g., Evans, 2007; Evans, Rich, Davies, & Allwood, 2008; Cale & Harris, 2005) after taking into account some of the issues highlighted earlier in this chapter. The earlier recommendations focus specifically on fitness, whereas the latter focus on monitoring within the curriculum more broadly, thus also covering the monitoring of health and physical activity. For ease, they have been combined and summarised here, as well as adapted and developed further in some parts. Collectively, the recommendations address the content, organisation and delivery of monitoring practices and the general principles, messages, attitudes, values and philosophy that teachers should strive to adopt and promote in their approach to monitoring (Cale & Harris, 2009b; Cale, Harris, & Chen, 2014; Cohen, Voss, & Sandercock, 2014).

Recommendations for Overall Approach to Fitness Monitoring

Fitness (or any) monitoring should neither dominate nor be conducted in isolation. Instead, it should be fully and appropriately integrated into a holistic health curriculum alongside coverage of a comprehensive range of relevant health-related content. Monitoring should be broad and process oriented and should focus on both health and activity. In addition, both teachers and pupils should approach monitoring with a critical attitude in order to raise their awareness of its advantages, disadvantages, limitations and potential issues.

More specifically, fitness monitoring should be used to promote health-related learning and to promote pupils' health, activity and fitness; therefore, it should focus less on outcomes (i.e., fitness results) and more on the process of monitoring and the associated learning (see the section titled Applying What You Learn From Physical Fitness Information). In addition, it should focus on the health-related components of fitness, primarily those that involve pupils in physical activity which develops: cardiorespiratory fitness, flexibility and muscular strength and endurance. Body composition can also be addressed if dealt with sensitively; however, because measures of body composition are static, they are less useful in promoting physical activity. Before undertaking fitness monitoring, consider carefully the purpose of the monitoring, the pupils involved, how they are likely to respond to and cope with fitness testing, and which tests and procedures are appropriate and inappropriate. If concerns arise, use alternative approaches.

Recommendations for Fitness Monitoring Methods, Tests and Procedures

Methods, tests and procedures should be selected carefully and sensitively and should be used in a manner that is inclusive and developmentally appropriate—for example, avoiding maximal tests, avoiding or modifying tests designed for adults, choosing measures carefully and offering choices of varying degrees of difficulty. The approaches you use should also be pupil centred (rather than activity centred), individualised and focused on personal improvement over time rather than on comparisons with others. These goals can be achieved by, for example, allowing pupils to work independently and direct practices, providing pupils with personalised baseline scores and feedback for improvement, and minimising the public and comparative nature of monitoring.

In order to conduct monitoring in a sensitive fashion, avoid focusing on or highlighting size and weight, which may dishearten, stigmatise or cause embarrassment or humiliation for some pupils (e.g., weighing and measuring to calculate BMI or using skinfold calipers in a public space). In addition, consider carefully whether some methods and procedures should be optional rather than compulsory. For example, weight and body composition can be addressed if dealt with sensitively, but public measurements of either should not be forced on pupils.

Addressing these concerns should enable fitness monitoring to be as positive, fun, varied, meaningful and relevant as possible. In order for pupils to build competence, confidence and a sense of control, they should be helped to understand and deal with their individual strengths and weaknesses in fitness and to feel good about themselves regardless of their size, weight or fitness (or health or activity) status. Fitness monitoring should never be administered at the expense of lowering an individual's self-concept or confidence.

Recommendations for Adopting Alternative Approaches to Fitness Monitoring

To ensure that fitness monitoring is positive, fun, varied, meaningful and relevant, we need to move it beyond traditional methods. It should include, for example, health and activity monitoring (see chapters 4 and 5), fitness monitoring options, home tasks, varied resources and equipment, self-monitoring and partner or peer (rather than whole-group) monitoring, and promotion and development of goal-setting skills. We also need to carefully consider the health information and messages provided alongside fitness monitoring, including their validity, how they may be received and interpreted, and how they may invite young people to feel about themselves and their bodies.

In addition, fitness monitoring results should be interpreted, explained and communicated in a meaningful way that helps pupils learn about maintaining and improving fitness. Pupils should be helped to review, interpret, and reflect on the scores and to understand the scores' limitations. The emphasis should be on encouraging pupils and helping them acquire and maintain fitness levels that are appropriate for their personal needs. If standards are used in interpreting scores, they should be explained and should be criterion referenced rather than normative. Criterion-referenced standards are achievable by the majority of pupils; they also reinforce the fitness–health link and the notion that most young people can be sufficiently fit and that a high level of fitness is not necessary for most individuals.

Whilst all pupils should be given constructive feedback, it is particularly important to provide individuals identified as 'very low fit' with appropriate, sensitive and personalized support, encouragement, guidance and targets. This feedback might involve suggesting activities or exercises they can undertake in their leisure time (at home or in the local community), communicating with parents, or, in extreme circumstances, recommending that they see their GP. Furthermore, we should recognise home influences on young people's health, activity and fitness levels in our evaluations and feedback and encourage parents (via letters, newsletters and invitations to events) to show interest in and support their children's health, physical activity and physical fitness.

Finally, we should exercise caution in deciding whether to implement test–retest monitoring procedures—for example, monitoring fitness at the beginning and again at the end of a unit of work or school year in order to identify changes. Programmes and units are often too short (six to eight weeks) to see measurable changes, and failure to do so could have a demotivating effect. The practice can also be time consuming and detract from learning time.

As noted in previous chapters, children learn about health, physical activity and healthy and active lifestyles within the curriculum. As part of this learning, it is relevant to increase children's awareness of their physical fitness levels and help them reflect on these levels. Practical ideas to help you deliver and promote learning through fitness monitoring are provided in the next section of this chapter and in the web resource. Specifically, the discussion here presents ideas for using physical fitness information to promote learning, whereas the web resource includes a selection of fitness tests considered appropriate for use in schools and during curriculum time to engage pupils in health-promoting physical activity. For each test and testing component, the resource provides an overview and general guidance, as well as pupil

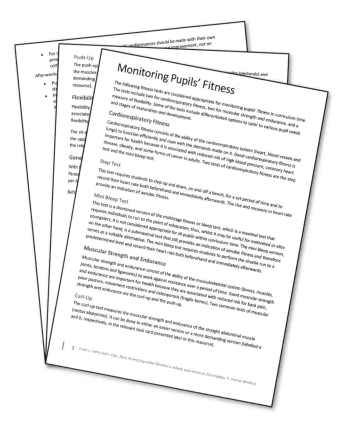

resources outlining specific procedures for the tests.

You can also choose from a number of formal and commercial test batteries for physical fitness, most of which measure common components of health-related fitness and include many of the same or similar tests, including some of those outlined earlier in this chapter and in the web resource. Thus, if you wish, you can adopt an existing commercial fitness test battery, either in its entirety or by selecting certain components of it. Alternatively, of course, you can develop your own tests and test batteries.

One well established test battery is Fitnessgram, which was developed by the Cooper Institute in the United States. This tool for physical fitness assessment, education and reporting addresses the five components of health-related fitness and uses criterion-referenced health standards, referred to as 'healthy fitness zones', to determine whether a pupil falls in the 'healthy zone'. Various iterations of Fitnessgram have been produced over the past 35 years, and the most recent version was released in 2017. The latest software provides individualised data and reports that summarise a child's performance on each component of fitness and gives opportunities for interaction with the data, as well as personalised

A NEW APPROACH TO FITNESS TESTING

For many years, the physical education department at Meadows Secondary School had conducted formal fitness monitoring of each year group at the start of the academic year. This process involved administering a standard battery of fitness tests designed to measure cardiorespiratory fitness, muscular strength and endurance, flexibility and body composition. However, the response from pupils to the monitoring was mixed, particularly for the multistage fitness or 'bleep' test, which was used as the measure of cardiorespiratory fitness with all pupils. Some of the more athletically able pupils were motivated by and enjoyed the test and saw it almost as a competitive event in which they openly tried to beat their peers. For others, the test had the opposite effect, and some pupils expended more energy in trying to avoid it than in taking it.

Similarly, teachers provided mixed views about the monitoring—particularly, the way in which it was implemented—and most were increasingly questioning its purpose and value. Key concerns raised by the physical education staff included the lack of learning and progression associated with the monitoring; the failure to analyse, interpret and use the data (the same tests were simply repeated each year); the negative attitudes towards the monitoring and the fact that many pupils saw no point in it; and the amount of time spent on the monitoring at the beginning of each year. All in all, many teachers felt that incorporating fitness monitoring at this time and in this way did not get the year off to the most positive and productive start.

> **Discussion points:** Does it surprise you to read of mixed views from pupils and teachers about the fitness testing in the PE programme? What are your own experiences and views of fitness testing in schools?

These concerns prompted the physical education department to conduct a thorough review of the fitness monitoring practices. The discussions were informed by afPE's health position paper (afPE, 2015a), as well as other fitness monitoring literature and recommendations, and resulted in a lively and healthy debate. In response, the department decided not to abandon fitness monitoring but to fundamentally change the way in which it was approached and delivered within the curriculum. For the first time, pupils were put at the heart of the monitoring, and careful consideration was given to their learning, experiences and needs.

Key learning outcomes were agreed on and embedded explicitly within the broader health curriculum alongside outcomes related to the broader monitoring of health and physical activity. These outcomes focused on developing pupils' knowledge and understanding of fitness monitoring (and fitness per se) and encouraging a critical attitude and approach towards monitoring; raising pupils' awareness of the advantages, disadvantages, limitations and potential issues associated with monitoring fitness; and ensuring an inclusive, individualised and empowering approach to monitoring. In short, the department shifted away from having pupils simply perform and towards helping them learn and develop broader knowledge and skills through fitness monitoring.

> **Discussion points:** Why did the department decide not to abandon fitness testing? What are your views on the department's shift in its approach to fitness testing?

Here are some of the practical ideas that the department developed and incorporated in order to support the new approach to fitness monitoring:

- Asking pupils to collect and critique articles, media reports and messages about fitness over the course of a general health unit

- Critiquing specific fitness tests with pupils in terms of their utility, validity, appropriateness and appeal for all young people

- Asking pupils to explore selected fitness tests to familiarise themselves with the tests and understand and develop their own (or a partner's) exercise technique

- Having pupils perform selected fitness tests of their choice, record the results, help administer the tests and provide feedback on their peers' technique

- Inviting pupils to analyse and interpret their own (or anonymous or fictitious) fitness data and consider what messages, advice and actions would be appropriate

- Organising and running a Get Fit and Active event to provide a range of fun fitness and physical activity opportunities for pupils to choose from, as well as various field-based measures of fitness, physical activity and health for them to participate in if they wish (and involving pupils in planning and delivering the event, including assisting with fitness and activity sessions and field-based fitness tests, with a focus on choice and engaging in various ways)

These ideas are in their first year of implementation, and the new approach will be reviewed in detail at the end-of-year physical education meeting. Whilst there will no doubt be some changes and developments based on lessons learned, indications to date suggest that the overall approach has been well received by both pupils and teachers and has led to enhanced learning by all.

> **Discussion points:** What advantages are offered by a pupil-centred, critical approach to fitness testing? What, if any, disadvantages might there be?

feedback, positive reinforcement and suggestions about how to promote and maintain good fitness based on the assessment results.

Applying What You Learn From Monitoring Physical Fitness

As with information about health and physical activity, physical fitness data can be used in various ways to promote learning. For example, fitness information can be used to prompt discussion, reflection and general questions about physical fitness and about the relationships between physical fitness, physical activity and lifestyles. Of course, the amount and depth of coverage should be adapted to pupils' ages and abilities. Here are some possible ways to use the data to facilitate pupils' learning:

- To enhance pupils' knowledge and understanding of physical fitness and the monitoring of physical fitness—for example, the components of health-related physical fitness and their importance to health; the value of monitoring physical fitness; methods of monitoring physical fitness; how to conduct and evaluate monitoring in general, as well as specific fitness tests and procedures; factors that influence physical fitness and scores on fitness tests; and how to improve physical fitness
- To develop pupils' awareness and knowledge of their own physical fitness (e.g., overall fitness levels, performance in certain components of fitness), their self-evaluation skills (e.g., ability to understand and interpret fitness levels and factors that influence them) and their views and attitudes towards fitness monitoring (Sample questions to ask pupils are outlined in the web resource for this chapter under the heading Post-Monitoring Physical Fitness Questions.)
- To facilitate pupils' goal setting and self-monitoring of physical fitness—for example, using the information as the basis for setting realistic goals to maintain or, if appropriate, increase their physical fitness

- To diagnose pupils' fitness needs for individual exercise prescription as applicable based on their current physical fitness levels and the extent to which they are meeting particular standards or norms
- To promote broader and more transferable skills in pupils (e.g., independent inquiry, critical reflection, problem solving, self-management) and cross-curricular skills and links between subjects (e.g., physical education, numeracy, science)

The information you gain from fitness monitoring will enhance your understanding of your pupils' physical fitness levels, their responses to fitness monitoring and testing, and their fitness ambitions. For example, you can use the information to inform both the curriculum and the content, nature, organisation and extent of any monitoring you decide to use in the future.

Summary

Monitoring children's physical fitness is commonplace in schools but remains controversial. Reasons for monitoring children's physical fitness in schools include promoting physical activity; enhancing learning and positive attitudes; and developing pupils' skills in goal setting, self-monitoring and self-testing. Children's physical fitness can be monitored in schools through field-based tests of health-related fitness. Your decisions about fitness monitoring should be informed by a critique of fitness monitoring, which will help you address issues related to the purpose and implementation of monitoring, as well as the interpretation and use of monitoring data.

If fitness monitoring is used appropriately, subjected to informed critique and incorporated as just one component of a broad and holistic health education programme, then it can serve as a valuable component of the curriculum and play a role in supporting healthy lifestyles and physical activity. Recommendations, guidelines and practical ideas are available to help you implement fitness monitoring and realise its potential to facilitate pupils' learning. With this guidance and support, you can adopt a healthy, activity-promoting approach to fitness monitoring.

PART III

Health-Related Learning in Physical Education

Involving All Children in Healthy, Active Lifestyles

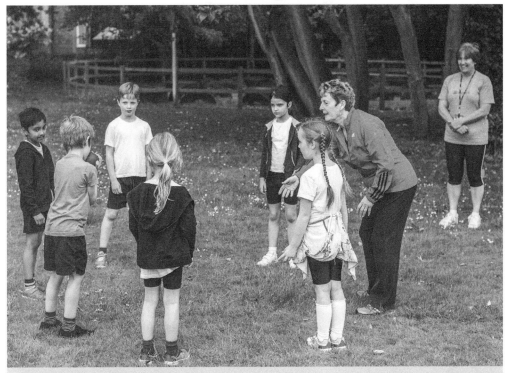

Chapter Objectives

After reading this chapter, you will be able to

- ▶ explain the rationale for involving all children in healthy, active lifestyles;
- ▶ identify the general philosophy, key principles and selected strategies for involving children of all abilities in physical activity;
- ▶ understand general information about common health conditions in young people (including asthma, diabetes and obesity) that is relevant to the promotion of healthy, active lifestyles; and
- ▶ apply general and specific practical recommendations for involving young people with asthma, diabetes and obesity in physical activity.

Given the established health benefits of physical activity and the fact that some children, including those with disabilities and medical conditions, face more barriers and challenges to participation than do others, this chapter focuses on helping *all* young people to lead healthy, active lifestyles. The chapter considers the rationale, philosophy and key principles underpinning an equitable approach to the promotion of physical activity and pays special attention to recommendations and strategies for involving young people with conditions including asthma, diabetes and obesity in physical activity.

Rationale for Involving All Children in Healthy, Active Lifestyles

Chapter 1 provides the rationale for promoting healthy, active lifestyles among children and an overview of the many benefits of physical activity for young people's physical, psychological and social health. This rationale and these benefits hold true for all young people, but engaging in appropriate physical activity may be particularly important and beneficial for some youngsters, such as those with particularly low self-esteem, physical competence or confidence; those who are overweight or obese; and those with other common medical conditions. Specific benefits of physical activity for children who have asthma or diabetes or who are obese are considered later in the chapter. In addition, in addressing the issue of 'striving to "include" in physical education and sport', Fitzgerald (2011, p. 158) identifies benefits beyond those associated with physical health and cognitive and psychological factors. These benefits include opportunities for young people to develop social skills and friendships, experience decreased isolation, develop higher expectations, meet more demanding challenges and enhance their appreciation of difference and equity.

All of these benefits aside, inclusive education is also enshrined in both national and international legislation. Therefore, schools have not only a moral and social obligation but also a legal one to promote inclusion, meet the needs of all pupils, remove barriers to learning and ensure an inclusive environment and curriculum. This obligation applies, of course, to the context of school physical activity and physical education, which should involve all children in physical activity through the provision of positive, relevant, meaningful and rewarding physical activity experiences. Indeed, such provision should be a fundamental goal of all schools.

Vickerman (2010) suggests that this obligation has led to a plethora of philosophies, policies and practices for promoting entitlement and access to physical education and opportunities for physical activity. In line with Vickerman's call for schools to meet their obligation to provide inclusive education, the following inclusive philosophy is advocated when promoting healthy, active lifestyles:

- Physical activity is for all.
- Physical activity is for life.
- Everyone can benefit from physical activity.
- Everyone has the right to positive physical activity experiences.
- Everyone can be good at physical activity.
- Excellence is maintaining an active way of life.

(adapted from Cale and Harris, 2009, p.117).

This philosophy can be implemented if schools and teachers critically examine their policies and practices for physical activity and physical education in light of their pupils and are committed and flexible in their approach. Speaking broadly about inclusive teaching and learning in physical education, Vickerman (2010) notes that the limiting factor for a child's inclusion lies with the teacher and that it is therefore important for schools to adopt flexible approaches rather than expecting all children to fit into existing structures. Vickerman goes on to identify the following critical factors for inclusion: high-quality learning and teaching; equipping of teachers with the necessary knowledge, skills and understanding to support a wide range of children's needs; and a positive school culture and willingness to modify and adapt activities and environments.

Vickerman (2010) also identified four key principles for maximising the potential of all children in physical education: entitlement, accessibility, inclusion and integrity. When applied to the context of healthy, active lifestyles, **entitlement** involves acknowledging the fundamental right of all children to access physical activity opportunities, whilst **accessibility** refers to teachers' responsibility to ensure that all pupils gain their full entitlement by devising effective strategies, adopting flexible approaches, and modifying and adapting activities as appropriate. **Inclusion** involves teachers first recognising the various physical activity needs of pupils and planning appropriately to meet them. And the principle of **integrity** is concerned with ensuring that any strategies used, and any modifications or adaptions made, are of equal worth and not patronising or tokenistic. In this regard, it is recommended that you consult with pupils and involve them in decision making.

Strategies for Involving All Children in Healthy, Active Lifestyles

Having considered the general philosophy and key principles of involving all children in physical activity, let us now consider strategies for supporting the involvement of all children. In order to succeed, efforts to empower young people to participate in healthy, active lifestyles must include three key elements: appropriate content, appropriate context and effective pedagogy (Elbourn & James, 2013). Appropriate content is safe, explicit, progressive, relevant, well informed, inclusive, exciting and fun. Appropriate context, in turn, consists of a range of activities through which healthy, active lifestyles can be promoted—for example, a variety of games and dance or gymnastics activities, or a range of fitness or exercise activities (e.g., aerobics, circuits). Effective pedagogy is, among other things, personalised, enabling and collaborative; moreover, it facilitates informed decision making and uses active learning strategies.

Content and Context

It may seem obvious that in order to involve all young people in physical activity, we must provide content that is safe, explicit, progressive, relevant, well informed, inclusive, exciting and fun. However, many of the physical activity opportunities provided in schools—and, notably, within physical education—are perceived by many pupils as traditional, irrelevant, boring and far from fun. For example, physical education continues to be dominated by a traditional sporting model that focuses on sport techniques, competitive sport and team games (Tannehill, 2012; Green, 2009; Kirk, 2010). Although this

model may be attractive for some, overemphasising it may turn many pupils off and leave the needs of many individuals unmet. In fact, the relevance and appeal of competitive sport and team games have been questioned for some time (Green, 2004; Fox & Harris, 2003; Haerens, Kirk, Cardon, & De Bourdeaudhuij, 2011) on the basis that they fail to acknowledge young people's leisure lifestyles as well as trends towards a wider range of noncompetitive recreational activities in informal, individual and small-group settings (Green, 2004).

Clearly, current participatory trends need to be reflected in the physical activity opportunities provided to pupils. In this respect, we need to take a broad approach to teaching about healthy, active lifestyles that provides a range of physical activities and focuses on pupils' development in the cognitive, psychomotor, behavioural and affective domains (Harris, 2000). In other words, we need an approach that both develops pupils' knowledge, understanding and competence in a range of physical activities and contexts and promotes positive attitudes towards and participation in physical activity. Recreational activities that may be attractive and relevant to pupils include swimming, cycling, dance, walking, hiking, jogging and fitness activities (e.g., skipping, aerobics, circuits, step, Pilates, boxercise, Zumba, spin, aquatics and yoga).

When choosing and delivering opportunities for physical activity, ask the following questions:

- Why am I choosing this activity?
- Is it relevant and meaningful to my pupils?
- Is it accessible?
- Are any pupils likely to be marginalised?
- Would any other activities be more inclusive and engaging?

Pedagogy

Regardless of the content and context, involving all pupils in healthy, active lifestyles also demands careful consideration of how physical activity is taught—that is, of pedagogy. Clearly, the delivery needs to be of high quality and marked by caring teaching strategies; it should also be grounded in a practical knowledge base and involve enjoyable, positive and meaningful physical activity experiences (Fox & Harris, 2003). Efforts to implement this sort of teaching, however, have encountered challenges. For one thing, limitations have been recognised in the pedagogy traditionally applied to teaching about active lifestyles such as an over-emphasis on testing and training; furthermore, knowledge about effective PE-for-health pedagogies has been identified as a significant gap in the field (Armour & Harris, 2013; Haerens et al., 2011). Indeed, in contrast to the considerable interest expressed in developing health-focused curriculum activities, less attention has been paid to developing effective pedagogies (Armour & Harris, 2013). In the prevailing or traditional pedagogical approach, the drivers are curriculum, programmes and activities rather than the needs of learners. In contrast, effective PE-for-health pedagogies put pedagogy and learners' needs at the core (Armour & Harris, 2013).

Given the lack of knowledge about appropriate pedagogies, it is perhaps not surprising that concerns have been raised over the delivery of education related to healthy, active lifestyles, both in schools generally and in physical education in particular. Just as concerns have been raised about the content of physical activity offered to pupils, questions have also been asked about teachers' ability and effectiveness in delivering that content and about the level of emphasis placed on that delivery. More specifically, teachers have been criticised for adopting an approach that emphasises sport, performance and fitness (Alfrey, Cale, & Webb, 2012; Harris & Leggett, 2015a, 2015b; Puhse et al., 2011) and for focusing on outcomes that are narrow. Such an approach is problematic because it is likely to highlight some pupils' inadequacies in the physical context, thus heightening their awareness that their physical performance does not match up with that of their peers and potentially turning them off of physical activity.

Thus, the key is to focus primarily on pupils and put their needs at the core, which begins with establishing what those needs are. Only when you understand young people's physical activity needs, interests, likes and dislikes—as well as their individual physical and psychological characteristics (e.g., level of fitness, physical limitations, self-esteem, confidence) and the barriers and other factors that influence their participation—are you likely to succeed at promoting and influencing their physical activity (Cale & Harris, 2009). Specifically, in order for pupils to feel successful in any activity, you must meet the following set of pupil needs: feeling competent, belonging, feeling useful, feeling potent and feeling optimistic (Sagor, 2002, cited in Tannehill, 2012). In order

to meet these needs, you must understand young people and their physical activity behaviour (and experiences). And to do that, you must listen to, engage with and empower them, because they are the experts on themselves and should be given a voice (Cale, 2011).

Indeed, consulting with pupils and involving them in decision making is linked to the principle of integrity discussed earlier (Vickerman, 2010) and is now commonly advocated in physical activity and physical education contexts (MacPhail & Halbert, 2005; Tannehill, 2012; Vickerman, 2010). Consultation with pupils is viewed as a central success factor because it enables teachers and pupils to consider, at the planning stage, any differentiation that may be required (Vickerman, 2010). In fact, with respect to physical education, it has been proposed that young people should be involved more intimately in a 'negotiated curriculum' process that addresses both what is taught (i.e., content) and how it is taught (i.e., pedagogy) (Tannehill, 2012, p. 235) so that pupils become partners in the development of a fully inclusive curriculum. At the same time, teachers should not merely teach what pupils want but should find ways 'to pull them in, motivate them to persevere, and provide them with what is important, relevant, and worth their time and energy to master' (Tannehill, 2012, p. 237). In summary, it is important to work with rather than at young people in the physical activity context, to respect their voices, and to avoid a 'nannying' approach to promoting healthy, active lifestyles (Cale, 2011).

There is one final strategy for supporting the involvement of all pupils in physical activity linked to pedagogy—namely, to adopt a specific model of inclusion. Various such models exist, but two are considered particularly useful and practical: the inclusion spectrum and the STEP model.

Inclusion Spectrum

The **inclusion spectrum** is an activity-centred approach to the inclusion of pupils with various abilities in physical activity (Stevenson, 2009). Whilst it was originally developed and adopted in relation to people with disability, it promotes meaningful involvement of all young people (with or without disability) in physical activity. It is based on the social model of disability, which holds that barriers to young people's participation result not from individual characteristics but from attitudinal, economic and environmental factors.

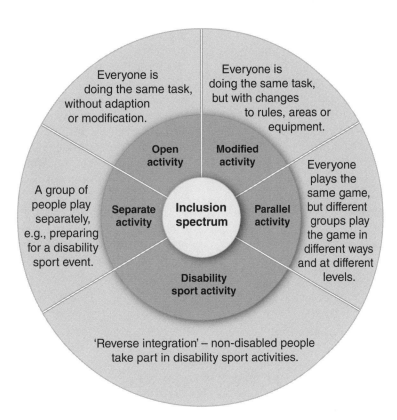

Figure 7.1 The inclusion spectrum.
Based on Stevenson 2009.

In practice, the inclusion spectrum provides a simple structure for inclusion that can be used flexibly with various activities and sports and with pupils of varying abilities to provide a range of options and delivery methods. It consists of five approaches to delivering physical activity that are arranged in a continuum of participation; each approach is designed to empower, deliver and encourage full participation of all young people (see figure 7.1).

Here are the five approaches of the inclusion spectrum.

1. **Open:** All pupils do the same activity without adaption or modification or in their own way without conditions. For example, this approach might include simple warm-up or cool-down activities, inclusive games, or continuous activity that all pupils can perform and in which individual differences are not so obvious.

2. **Modified:** Everyone does the same activity with adaptions to appropriately challenge and support the inclusion of all pupils. For example, adaptions might be made to the rules, space or equipment in order to facilitate all pupils' participation. (For

more details, see the following discussion of the STEP model.)

3. **Parallel:** Pupils are grouped according to ability, and everyone does the same activity but each pupil performs at an appropriate level. For example, this approach might involve using different versions of the same activity, game or exercise (e.g., standing or seated volleyball; box or full push-up); a range of small-sided activities; or ability-matched zones within a larger activity.

4. **Separate:** A pupil or group of pupils does a purposefully planned activity that is different from what the rest of the class does— for example, practising an individual or specific skill or preparing for a particular group or team event.

5. **Disability sport:** This approach includes aspects of physical activity based on disability sport. This 'reverse integration' provides specific opportunities for pupils with disability and new challenges for pupils without disability. Examples include the disability sports of boccia, goalball and sitting volleyball.

The appeal of the inclusion spectrum lies in its simplicity and its underpinning by the social model of disability. However, little research has been carried out on its effectiveness, and it is subject to some limitations. For example, it has been suggested that the model does little to question prevailing 'normative practices' (or to take teachers and coaches forward to a more complex and demanding understanding of inclusion) and that implementing it effectively requires teachers to reinterpret and fully apply the philosophical principles that underpin it (Fitzgerald, 2011, 2012).

STEP Model

Linked to the inclusion spectrum, the **STEP model** is another simple framework for facilitating all pupils' involvement in physical activity. The model holds that all pupils can be included and challenged to progress if teachers appropriately modify their delivery of activities. Changes can be made in one or more of four areas indicated by the STEP acronym: space, task, equipment and people (see table 7.1). In this context, the space is where the activity happens, the task is what happens, the equipment is what is used, and the people are those who are involved. The STEP model requires teachers to address each of these areas in the planning stage and ask the following question: How can I change the space, task, equipment, or people (or some combination of these factors) to involve all pupils?

ACTIVITY FOR ALL

A primary school in the Midlands decided to focus on improving the health of its population by reviewing the activity opportunities available to pupils during breaks and lunchtimes. School staff and governors concluded that current activity opportunities were too limited and therefore were accessed by only a minority of the pupils (mostly those who were healthier and more fit, able and active). In response, the staff were particularly keen to ensure that every child, including those with disabilities and medical conditions (e.g., asthma, diabetes, obesity) could participate in activity opportunities.

To achieve this goal, the school decided to offer pupils a mixture of structured and unstructured activities during breaks and lunchtimes on Mondays, Wednesdays and Fridays. They also decided to permit pupils to borrow equipment (e.g., balls, hoops, cones, skipping ropes); to provide volunteer supervision by teaching assistants, parents and older 'active buddy' pupils for children undertaking playground activities (e.g., hopscotch, throwing balls against targets on walls or the ground); and to organise activities, such as walking (or jogging or skipping) around a series of cones, throwing beanbags and jumping over a series of low hurdles.

Discussion points: Why do you think that both structured and unstructured activities were offered? What are your views on involving older 'active buddy' pupils in this initiative?

The activities were offered during the entire summer term and resulted in an increased proportion of children being active during breaks and lunchtimes. Children enjoyed the range of activities on offer and the freedom to borrow equipment to make up and play their own activities. Teachers considered the initiative successful in engaging most of the children with specific disabilities and health conditions (who previously had been inactive during breaks and lunchtimes). Many parents of these children praised the initiative, and some supported it by volunteering to assist on particular days of the week.

Discussion points: Why do you think that children with specific health conditions engaged with the initiative? What are the benefits of involving parents in the initiative? What safeguarding concerns need to be addressed when involving parents?

After the initiative was reviewed at a governors' meeting, the school decided to continue it during the following autumn term and to encourage involvement by more parents and more of the older pupils. The governors also decided to raise funds to pay for additional markings on the walls and grounds of the school and for additional modified equipment, such as low hurdles and soft javelins.

TABLE 7.1   Options for Modifying Physical Activities Within the STEP Framework

Space	Where?	
	• Size of playing area (more or less space) • Distance to be travelled • Use of zoned activity or playing areas • Targets nearer or further away • Level (height; e.g., floor-based or seated versus ambulant)	
Task	What?	
	• Easier or harder tasks or versions of activities • Specific and different roles (e.g., coach, official, performer) • Rotating roles • Different rules (e.g., allowing different places to start) • Different ways of taking part (e.g., seated, standing, lying) • Different targets	
Equipment	What is used?	
	Type	Characteristic
	• Balls • Bats • Rackets • Cones or markers • Beanbags • Scarves • Mats	• Size • Shape • Weight • Softness • Colour • Texture
People	With whom?	
	Type of participation	Roles, groupings and space
	• Independent • In pairs, groups or teams • With friends • With learning support assistant	With: • Different or same roles • Different or same ability • Different or same size In: • Own space • Large space • Small space • Restricted space • Open space

Involving Children With Common Health Conditions in Physical Activity

Throughout this book, we highlight the importance of promoting healthy, active lifestyles to all young people. For young people with certain common health conditions, however, physical activity offers particular benefits. Furthermore, as noted earlier, schools have a legal responsibility to ensure that all pupils have full access to education, which includes school physical activity and physical education opportunities. Indeed, it is now statutory in England to make arrangements to support pupils with medical conditions, and statutory guidance is available to ensure that such pupils can access and enjoy the same opportunities as any other child, play a full and active role in school life, remain healthy and achieve their potential (see Department for Education, 2015).

In that context, this section of the chapter examines how to involve young people with the following health conditions in physical activity: asthma, diabetes and obesity. The section begins by presenting key background information about each condition, such as prevalence, symptoms and benefits of physical activity in relation to the condition. Alongside the benefits, however, we must consider some important sensitivities likely to affect an individual's ability to participate, as well as his or her enjoyment of and attitude towards participation. These sensitivities are taken into account in practical recommendations for involving youngsters with such conditions in physical activity.

Asthma

Asthma is a common condition affecting the airways, or tubes, that carry air in and out of the lungs. When a person with asthma comes into contact with a trigger, the airways get irritated and become narrower, thus making it difficult for the person to breathe and leading to symptoms such as chest tightness, wheezing, coughing and shortness of breath (British Heart Foundation, 2011; Asthma UK, 2016b). Asthma affects as many as 334 million people of all ages in all parts of the world; more specifically, the latest International Study of Asthma and Allergies in Childhood (ISAAC) survey found that 14 percent of the world's children were likely to have had asthmatic symptoms in the preceding year (Global Asthma Network, 2014). In the United Kingdom, asthma is reported to be the most common long-term medical condition among children, affecting more than 1.1 million youngsters, which translates to about 1 in every 10 children and about 2 pupils per school class (British Lung Foundation, 2016).

Not all young people with asthma experience all of the symptoms; moreover, the severity and duration of symptoms vary, both between individuals and between attacks in the same person. Youngsters with mild asthma may experience symptoms only with certain triggers, whereas those with severe asthma may experience permanent narrowing of the airways.

Major asthma triggers include the following:

- Viral infections, especially of the respiratory tract
- Irritants, such as dust, air pollution, fumes and smoke (including cigarette smoke)

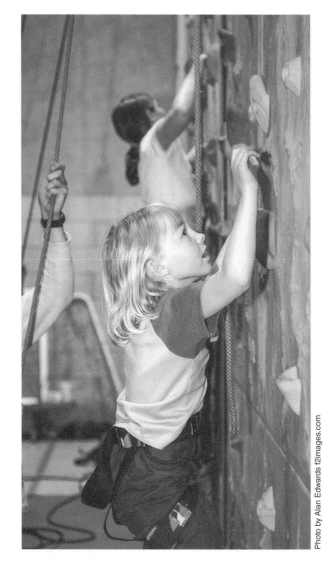

Children with particular needs can be introduced to a range of physical activities as part of a school's physical education curriculum and extra-curricular programme.

- Allergens, such as dust mites, pollen, bird feathers and animal dander and secretions
- Weather changes, such as cold winds, thunderstorms and decreases in temperature
- Expressions of emotion, such as amusement (via laughter), anger, fear and stress
- Exercise or other physical activity, particularly continuous aerobic exercise

(British Heart Foundation, 2011, p. 38–39).

If a child's asthma is often triggered by exercise, then the condition may not be as well controlled as it could be. Moreover, if exercise is the only trigger, then the child may have exercise-induced asthma, which involves the usual asthma symptoms but begins during or after participation in exercise or physical activity. It can become more severe about 15 minutes after exercise ends, then gradually improve.

It is not fully understood how physical activity triggers asthma symptoms, but some believe it is associated with breathing in cold, dry air more quickly and forcefully than when not exercising (British Heart Foundation, 2011). In some people, the airways are sensitive to changes in temperature and humidity and react by getting narrower. The treatment for exercise-induced asthma is the same as for other kinds of asthma, and young people with this form of asthma can still take part in physical activity, provided that they learn how to reduce their risk of experiencing symptoms and how to manage symptoms when they do occur (Asthma UK, 2016a).

For children with asthma, physical activity provides benefits over and above the general ones highlighted in chapter 1. For example, the British Heart Foundation (2011) and Asthma UK (2016a) note that physical activity can

- lead to improved cardiorespiratory fitness (and reduced breathlessness at a given exercise intensity), thereby providing extra stamina for coping with asthma during everyday activities;

- improve respiratory muscle strength and lung capacity, which exert both short- and long-term positive effects on breathing and asthma control;

- help young people maintain or attain a healthy weight, which helps reduce the risk of asthma attacks and other asthma symptoms and may reduce the need for medication to control asthma;

- boost the immune system, thus making asthma less likely to be triggered by coughs and colds; and

- positively influence mood (i.e., reduce stress and depression) and thereby reduce the risk of stress-induced asthma.

Diabetes

Diabetes is a condition in which the amount of glucose (sugar) in the blood is too high, either because the pancreas does not produce any or enough insulin or because the insulin produced does not work properly (Diabetes UK, 2016). Insulin helps the glucose move from the blood into the body's cells to be used as energy; without it, the body cannot use glucose. Diabetes can be either type 1 or type 2. In type 1, the immune system attacks healthy body tissue in the pancreas, thus making it unable to produce insulin and leaving the body unable to move glucose out of the bloodstream and into cells. This type of diabetes is often inherited and is not caused by unhealthy lifestyle choices. Type 2 diabetes, on the other hand, occurs when the body does not produce enough insulin to function properly or when the body's cells do not react to insulin; in either case, glucose stays in the blood and is not used as fuel for energy. Type 2 diabetes is often associated with obesity and unhealthy lifestyle choices and tends to be diagnosed in older adults.

In the United Kingdom, about 31,500 young people live with diabetes, and the vast majority have type 1 (Diabetes UK, 2015). In addition, according to an international league table compiled by Diabetes UK and based on estimates from the International Diabetes Federation, the United Kingdom has the world's fifth-highest rate of diagnosis for type 1 diabetes in children aged up to 14 years. Type 2 diabetes was first diagnosed in overweight girls of Pakistani, Indian or Arabic origin in the United Kingdom in 2000 and in white adolescents in 2002, and the number of young people with this condition is increasing as more become overweight and obese (British Heart Foundation, 2011). As of now, there is no cure for diabetes, but both types can be managed and treated. Treatment for type 1 diabetes involves taking insulin, either via injection or via an insulin pump; in addition, eating a healthy diet and getting regular physical activity are advised for overall good health (British Heart Foundation, 2011). Treatment for Type 2 diabetes ranges from lifestyle adjustments to tablet medication and injections (British Heart Foundation, 2011).

Here are the main symptoms of diabetes in young people:

- Passing more urine than normal
- Increased thirst
- Extreme tiredness
- Weight loss

These symptoms are sometimes referred to as the four Ts: toilet, thirsty, tired and thinner (Diabetes UK, 2014).

Physical activity provides a number of benefits that are particularly relevant for young people with diabetes, including the following:

- Helps young people maintain a healthy weight, which in turn helps control their diabetes.

- Helps the body use insulin more efficiently and therefore may help reduce the amount taken and improve overall diabetes management.

- Helps lower blood-sugar levels, which may also help reduce the amount of insulin taken.

- Improves overall diabetes control and helps prevent some of the complications associated with diabetes in later life (British Heart Foundation, 2011, p. 109; Diabetes UK, 2016).

Obesity

The World Health Organisation (2016) classifies individuals with a body mass index (BMI) of 25 or more as overweight and those with a BMI of 30 or more as obese. BMI is determined by dividing the square of an individual's height in metres into his or her weight in kilograms. To account for growth patterns by age and gender, a child's BMI is compared with BMI centiles in published growth charts; children above the 95th centile are classified as obese (HM Government, 2016). Using BMI as a measure of obesity is subject to some limitations as it does not, for example, take account of different stages of physical maturity, and the classification of obesity in children is controversial as they are still growing and have not reached full physical maturity. Despite these caveats, BMI is used as a measure of obesity as it is relatively simple and low in cost.

As noted in chapter 1, concerns over the increased prevalence of obesity among children and adolescents have been raised in recent decades. In fact, the World Health Organisation (2016) has reported that the number of infants and young children considered overweight or obese increased by 10 million globally between 1990 and 2013, to a current total of 42 million. Recent figures in England indicate that nearly a third of children aged 2 to 15 years are overweight or obese and that the obesity rate is 16 percent among boys and 15 percent among girls (Health and Social Care Information Centre, 2015b).

Alarmingly, nearly 80 percent of children who are obese in their teens are likely to remain obese as adults (National Institute for Health and Care Excellence, 2015).

In considering these statistics, we must recognise that obesity and overweight differ from each other and that combining them (as is typically done) inflates the figures and thus distorts the picture to some degree. As explained by Cale and Harris (2009), obesity is a clinical health condition, whereas overweight is not; moreover, whilst overweight can lead to obesity, it generally does not. Nonetheless, a significant number of young people are obese and have difficulty attaining and maintaining a healthy body weight. In addition, many of the issues and benefits of physical activity apply equally to both obesity and overweight. Therefore, both are considered here.

Contributions to obesity can come from a variety of factors. Whilst genetics can make some young people more susceptible than others, this factor alone is not sufficient; nor does it constitute the main cause. Both obesity itself and the increase in obesity more likely result from behavioural factors (i.e., changes in physical activity, diet and eating patterns) and environmental factors (e.g., access to physical activity opportunities, increased availability and affordability of certain types of food) (Cale & Harris, 2009, p. 140). Thus obesity is undoubtedly facilitated by **obesogenic environments**— that is, environments that encourage people to eat unhealthily and fail to exercise sufficiently. Examples include places that encourage driving rather than walking, buildings with lifts and escalators prominently sited and stairs hidden away, and public places dominated by shops that sell calorie-dense foods.

Such environments encourage people to live with an unhealthy energy balance. The energy balance equation explains the relationship between energy intake (what we eat and drink, or calories consumed), energy expenditure (what we expend in daily living and physical activity, or calories burned) and body weight:

Energy intake = energy expenditure → stable weight

Energy intake > energy expenditure → weight gain

Energy intake < energy expenditure → weight loss

Put simply, then, individuals gain weight when their energy intake exceeds their energy expenditure. However, energy imbalance is not a straightforward physical issue, because relationships with food and drink are complex and are affected by behaviour, environment, genetics and culture.

Young people who are overweight or obese can gain numerous benefits from physical activity; specifically, it can

- increase **lean body mass** (total mass or weight minus body fat) and **energy expenditure** (energy or calories used for functions such as breathing, digestion and movement), thereby helping achieve and maintain **energy balance** (equilibrium between energy intake and energy expenditure) and preventing weight gain;

- improve a young person's metabolic profile (e.g., produce favourable changes in blood cholesterol levels and increase insulin sensitivity);

- help protect against or manage other health problems and conditions associated with obesity (e.g., high blood pressure, type 2 diabetes, asthma);

- improve psychological well-being and help young people feel good about themselves and

- help prevent or reverse the downward spiral into inactivity due to associated health difficulties and complications that make participation more difficult (British Heart Foundation, 2011; Cale & Harris, 2009).

Recommendations for Involving Children With Asthma, Diabetes and Obesity in Physical Activity

Recommendations for involving young people with asthma, diabetes and obesity in physical activity can be either condition specific or general—that is, applying to all pupils with health conditions. This section begins with general recommendations, then offers condition-specific recommendations that address factors such as clothing, preparation, organisation, environment, and the nature (i.e., type, duration and intensity) of physical activities. All of the recommendations presented here have been informed by or adapted or developed from recommendations published previously by various authors and organisations (e.g., Association for Physical Education, 2016; Asthma UK, 2016a; British Heart Foundation, 2011; Cale & Harris, 2009, 2013; Department of Health, 2007; Diabetes UK 2014, 2016; Evans, 2007; National Institute for Clinical Excellence, 2006; National Institute for Health and Care Excellence, 2015).

Collectively, these recommendations will help you respond appropriately to pupils with health conditions; promote appropriate messages; and enable all pupils to engage in safe, effective and enjoyable physical activity both within and beyond school. All of the recommendations relate to physical activity or physical education; they do *not* touch on general guidance or requirements for supporting pupils with medical conditions across the whole school (e.g., developing individual health care plans or equivalents, consulting with other professionals and parents, managing medicines, keeping records, establishing emergency procedures). You should, of course, follow whole-school policies, practices and requirements in line with statutory duty and guidance, as applicable (see for example, Department for Education, 2015).

Here are the general recommendations:

- Pupils should be encouraged to adopt and maintain regular physical activity both in school (in both curricular and extracurricular physical education) and beyond school; they should also be made aware of the importance and specific benefits of physical activity for them.

- Pupils and their health conditions should not be seen as problems. In fact, provided that their conditions are appropriately controlled and managed, young people with asthma, diabetes or obesity should be able to readily engage in and reap the benefits of regular physical activity.

- Most young people are aware of their own capabilities and limitations in the realm of physical activity and know how to manage their conditions, especially in the case of older pupils. Communicate and consult with pupils to establish what they can and cannot do in terms of participation, as well as what they enjoy doing; involve them in decision making. Wherever possible, physical activity opportunities and guidance should be personalised to pupils' abilities, the severity of their conditions, their fitness levels or other limitations, and their preferences. This personalisation helps ensure that opportunities are accessible and appropriate and that pupils' experiences are safe and enjoyable.

- Pupils should refrain from participating in physical activity if they feel unwell, and they should stop physical activity if they feel pain, weakness or dizziness.

- Young people with health conditions may lack self-esteem, confidence and a sense of control; they may also experience self-consciousness, embarrassment or feelings of alienation. However, a sensitive, caring and inclusive approach can help them feel confident, valued, accepted and able to enjoy and achieve within the context.

- All pupils should be helped to feel good about themselves and their bodies; to understand and deal with their individuality, strengths and weaknesses; and to be proud of who they are. Pupils should be encouraged and helped to like themselves and their bodies and to celebrate being special. See the chapter 7 web resource for more information about how to involve children of all sizes in physical education and physical activity.

Involving Children of All Sizes in Physical Education and Physical Activity

Physical Activity's Contribution to Healthy Weight Management

Physical activity has the potential to reduce body fat in children and to provide a range of additional benefits such as improved skeletal health, increased self-confidence and improved social skills. Therefore, children of all shapes and sizes should be encouraged to be active. The shape children are in is more important than their body shape. Children should be encouraged to participate in as much routine activity as possible in order to increase their total energy expenditure (e.g. walking or cycling to school, using the stairs instead of the lift) and to reduce the amount of time they spend in sedentary activities (e.g. watching television, playing computer games and surfing the web).

Considerations for Involving Obese Children in Physical Education and Physical Activity

- Develop policies that are accommodating and sensitive to children's feelings about what they wear and about changing in front of others.
- Take care in selecting activities, tasks, positions and responsibilities allocated to pupils to reduce the risk of anyone feeling disheartened or embarrassed or being excluded or subject to teasing, ridicule or isolation from peers.
- Modify activities to accommodate individual body sizes and varying levels of exercise tolerance and movement efficiency (e.g. reducing the size of the playing area, increasing the number of players or performers, using equipment that is differently weighted or sized; performing low intensity, low impact versions of specific exercises).
- Incorporate activities that involve everyone (e.g., simple warm-ups, activities that involve social integration and interaction) to help children socialise and make friends.
- Vary activities frequently to avoid fatigue of the same muscle groups and joints.
- Encourage aerobic or continuous activity (of low to moderate intensity) which involves working large muscle groups for a sustained period of time and increases energy expenditure.
- Start with low intensity activity, then progress gradually to a maintenance level of low to moderate intensity; emphasise a gradual increase in the difficulty, duration and frequency rather than in the intensity.
- Encourage low-impact activities (e.g., walking, stepping) and non-weight-bearing activities (e.g., swimming, aqua aerobics, seated aerobics, seated multigym work, cycling, indoor rowing) that put less stress on the bones and joints and are easier and more comfortable to perform.
- Encourage activities that promote and improve muscular strength (and increase fat-free mass and muscle tone) and muscular endurance; these can also improve balance and coordination, making it easier to carry out everyday tasks and lead a more active lifestyle.
- Incorporate activities that promote and improve balance and posture such as dance and gymnastics activities and circuits including exercises for the postural muscles.
- Include games activities as they typically involve intermittent or short bouts of physical activity and include rest periods; however, ensure that they are managed sensitively to ensure that all pupils are included and accepted within the group.

1   From J. Harris and L. Cale, 2019, *Promoting active lifestyles in schools web resource* (Champaign, IL: Human Kinetics).

Practical Recommendations for Children With Asthma

Pupils should be dressed appropriately for the activity and conditions. For example, cold weather is likely to trigger symptoms of asthma because it can irritate sensitive airways. When it is cold, therefore, pupils with asthma should cover their chest and throat and possibly wear a scarf around the nose. When it is particularly cold, and where possible, exercising indoors may be advisable. In addition, prior to any energetic activity, sufficient time should be allowed for a thorough warm-up in which the intensity is increased gradually in order to reduce the risk of exercise-induced asthma. The warm-up should last at least 10 minutes and involve activities in which the intensity can be controlled by the individual. Afterwards, give the pupil sufficient time to cool down by gradually reducing the intensity of activity. This approach slows the change in temperature of the air entering the airways.

Individuals with asthma are also likely to fare better with interval-type or intermittent physical activities (i.e., those that require bursts of activity interspersed with activity of a lower intensity) than with continuous or endurance activities. Examples of interval-type activities include relay races, short sprints with recovery periods, chasing and tag games, and more formal team and individual games. Such activities can help pupils develop aerobic endurance, thereby strengthening their respiratory muscles and improving their cardiopulmonary function and general physical condition. Specific activities that may work well include racket-and-net games (e.g., badminton, table tennis, possibly short tennis) and striking and fielding games (e.g., cricket, rounders). Racket-and-net games involve less distance to cover and can generally be played at a slower pace and lower intensity. Striking-and-fielding games include short breaks following bouts of activity, and the pace and positions can be altered to suit various needs and abilities. Some pupils may struggle to participate in full team games, in which case you can use modified versions informed by the STEP model outlined earlier (e.g., reducing the playing area or putting more players on each team); for further possible modifications, see table 7.1.

In contrast, continuous physical activities (e.g., running for more than six minutes) require extended energy output and are much more likely to trigger exercise-induced asthma. Therefore, they may need to be avoided in some cases, particularly in cold weather. If continuous activities are included, they should be performed at a gentle pace, and the duration should be increased gradually. In particular, swimming is associated with better lung function and a lower risk of asthma symptoms because of the warm and humid air and is therefore considered to be one of the best forms of physical activity for individuals with asthma. Gymnastics and dance activities are also suitable for young people with asthma as they lend themselves to brief bursts of activity of varied intensity, make less aerobic demand, and are therefore to be encouraged. If you are looking to involve pupils in outdoor and adventurous activities, take care because some of these activities may cause asthma symptoms due to factors such as the environment, the weather or pupils' emotional state arising from the activity. Moreover, Asthma UK (2016b) recommends that young people with asthma seek medical advice from a GP before taking part in any adventure sport.

Practical Recommendations for Children With Diabetes

Pupils whose diabetes is controlled should be able to take part in any form of physical activity, and a variety of activities should be encouraged. These pupils should, however, start slow and gradually increase the amount of physical activity that they perform within a single session. Aerobic or continuous activities are recommended—for example, walking, jogging, cycling, swimming, skipping and dancing—because they allow pupils to control the duration and intensity which helps them manage their response to the increased demand on their bodies.

In order to allow pupils with diabetes to plan appropriately, they should be informed in advance about the nature of the physical activity to be performed (e.g., duration and intensity). A child's preparations for activity will vary depending on when the child last took insulin; the timing, type and duration of the activity; when the child last ate; and the child's blood glucose level (Diabetes UK [2014] recommends that young people check their blood glucose level before participating in any physical activity). For example, planning might involve eating a snack beforehand, having snacks available, or altering an insulin dose. Be sure to check that pupils with diabetes have prepared themselves as needed before they take part in any physical activity. Also encourage them

to recognise how they respond to different types of physical activity and to use that knowledge to make informed adjustments to their food and insulin, with support as appropriate.

Pupils with diabetes should also be encouraged to eat and drink both during and after physical activity in order to replace the glucose (energy) used; this is especially true if the activity is strenuous or prolonged (60 minutes or longer). In terms of liquid consumption, water or sugar-free squash is fine for activity lasting less than an hour, but for longer activities fruit juice or sugar-containing squash or drinks are recommended. After swimming, pupils may need to eat more carbohydrates than normal because extra energy is likely to be needed in order to maintain body temperature.

If a pupil's blood glucose level is too low (i.e., below 4 millimoles per litre, or mmol/L), then he or she should not be physically active until the level has been treated—for example, by consuming fast carbohydrate in the form of biscuits or a sugary drink followed by long-acting carbohydrate from a sandwich, banana or cereal bar. The goal is to achieve a blood sugar level of 5 mmol/L or more before the pupil begins any planned activity in order to reduce the risk of an incident of hypoglycaemia. Similarly, if a pupil's blood glucose level is too high (i.e., 14 mmol/L or more), then the pupil should wait until the level comes down before taking part in physical activity. The reason is that exercise triggers the release of stored glycogen from the liver, which causes blood glucose levels to rise; this process may continue if insulin levels are inadequate and the muscles are unable to use the glucose. Although relatively rare, this development can cause exercise-induced hyperglycaemia.

Practical Recommendations for Children Who Are Overweight or Obese

For these pupils, careful consideration must be given to policies related to kit, clothing, changing and showering. These policies should be sensitive to pupils' feelings about what they wear and about changing in front of others; where possible, such policies should also be flexible and accommodating. For example, private changing facilities should be provided where possible and pupils should be permitted to wear clothing in which they feel most comfortable (e.g., tracksuit bottoms; T-shirts for swimming).

In terms of activities, incorporate physical activities that involve everyone (e.g., simple warm-ups, circle or other games, activities that involve social integration and interaction) to help pupils socialise and make friends. Where possible, physical activities should be varied frequently to avoid overuse or fatigue of the same muscle groups and joints. Pupils should also be encouraged to incorporate variety when participating in physical activity on their own.

Pupils who are overweight or obese will find it particularly difficult and uncomfortable to participate in high-intensity, continuous activities (e.g., running and jumping), and such activities should not be forced on overweight or obese pupils. The reason is that obese children tend to have lower levels of fitness, especially cardiorespiratory fitness, than do their same-age peers of more typical weight. They are also more prone to overheating due to the insulating property of fat and therefore tend to have poor tolerance for exercise. To reduce the risk of overheating, pupils should be encouraged to drink water before, during and after physical activity.

The principal type of activity for overweight or obese pupils should be aerobic or continuous activity (of low to moderate intensity), which involves working the large muscle groups for a sustained period of time. This type of activity increases pupils' energy expenditure and helps improve their fitness and exercise tolerance. Pupils with larger bodies and more body weight may be less movement efficient in certain activities (e.g., running, balancing, rolling) and thus may find them particularly demanding. Therefore, physical activity may at first need to be of very low intensity, then progress gradually to a maintenance level of low to moderate intensity. Emphasise a gradual increase in the difficulty, duration and frequency rather than in the intensity.

Pupils who are overweight or obese are likely to struggle with managing their body weight and to have difficulty with activities that are high impact or require carrying or lifting the body—for example, running, jumping and taking weight on the hands. Obese children also face greater risk of orthopaedic injury (e.g., fracture) and may experience orthopaedic problems (e.g., knock knees, flat feet). Therefore, they should be encouraged to engage in low-impact activities (e.g., walking, stepping) and non-weight-bearing activities (e.g., swimming, aqua aerobics, seated aerobics, seated multigym work, cycling, indoor rowing) that put less stress on the bones and joints and are also easier and more comfortable to perform. Non-weight-bearing activities are particularly appropriate because the body weight is supported, thus making movement easier and reducing the risk of injury.

In addition, such pupils should be encouraged to engage in physical activities that promote and improve muscular strength (and increase fat-free mass and muscle tone) and muscular endurance. These activities also improve balance and coordination, thus making it easier for pupils to carry out everyday tasks and lead a more active lifestyle. Examples include climbing and swinging for younger pupils and circuits or resistance exercises for older age groups. If using fixed resistance equipment, however, all pupils should avoid intense or maximal resistance work. For specific guidelines on resistance training, consult *Safe Practice in Physical Education, School Sport and Physical Activity* from the Association for Physical Education (afPE) (2016).

Pupils who are overweight or obese may also have other orthopaedic problems, such as back pain and poor posture (e.g., slouching, rounded shoulders, excessive curving of the lower back). To address these issues, incorporate physical activities that promote and improve balance and posture wherever feasible. Possibilities include dance and gymnastics activities and circuits involving various exercises—for example, the flamingo balance or working postural muscles such as the shoulders (trapezius, rhomboids) and back (erector spinae) in shoulder squeezes and back lifts, respectively. Some pupils, particularly those who are severely obese, will likely have difficulty with floor-based activities and with moving from lying to upright positions; therefore, these activities may need to be avoided or minimised for obese pupils.

For most pupils who are obese, games are suitable and should be encouraged because they typically involve intermittent or short bouts of physical activity and include rest periods. However, they should be managed sensitively (especially team games) to ensure that all pupils are appropriately included and accepted within the group. To make appropriate modifications to games and activities, use the STEP model to accommodate individual body sizes and various levels of exercise tolerance and movement efficiency. Modifications might include, for example, reducing the size of the playing area, increasing the number of players or performers or using equipment that is differently weighted or differently sized.

Also take care in selecting the physical activities, tasks, positions and responsibilities allocated to pupils in order to reduce the risk of anyone feeling disheartened or embarrassed or being excluded or subject to teasing, ridicule or isolation from peers. For example, pupils should not be subjected to assault courses that involve squeezing through or jumping over equipment; unfair races (e.g., those in which some pupils are clearly advantaged by their physique); public displays; activities or games involving constant running or jumping; or routinely or frequently being assigned to inactive or lower-status roles or positions (e.g., scorer, goalkeeper, equipment helper). With these concerns in mind, and in the interest of safety, you should also carefully consider your grouping procedures. For example, weight and size should be taken into account when grouping pupils for partner or group tasks and activities (e.g., marking, defending or tackling in games; supporting or doing partner or group balancing in gymnastics). For these reasons, it is not recommended that you allow pupils to freely pick their own teams.

Some pupils demonstrate skill and aptitude for particular activities, especially in techniques involving small-muscle groups or activities or athletic events demanding muscular strength. Teachers should establish which activities their pupils show aptitude for and actively promote and encourage participation in these options. Pupils' achievements and successes in physical activity are likely to exert a positive influence on their confidence and self-esteem (which often pose challenges for youngsters) and therefore encourage them to continue participating. Pupils should also be encouraged to participate in as much routine physical activity as possible beyond school in order to increase their total energy expenditure—for example, walking or cycling to school or the shops, using the stairs instead of the lift, and assisting with tasks around the home (e.g., housework, gardening). At the same time, they should be encouraged to reduce the amount of time they spend in sedentary activities, such as watching television, playing computer or video games and surfing the web.

Summary

Whilst general health benefits of physical activity apply to all children, certain additional benefits apply to children with disabilities and specific health conditions such as asthma, diabetes and obesity. Inclusive education is enshrined in legislation and requires schools to involve all children in positive, relevant, meaningful and rewarding physical activity experiences. This requirement is underpinned by an inclusive philosophy, key principles (of entitlement, accessibility, inclusion and integrity), high-quality learning and teaching, commitment and a willingness to be flexible. In order to meet the goal of involving and empowering young people in healthy, active lifestyles, we must provide appropriate content in appropriate contexts through effective pedagogy. This work includes providing a range of physical activities in a range of contexts and adopting caring teaching strategies, pupil-centred approaches and specific models of inclusion.

Common health conditions in young people include asthma, diabetes and obesity. Each of these conditions is marked by certain triggers, causes, symptoms, complications and considerations. Fortunately, pupils with each condition can also benefit from physical activity. By implementing key recommendations for involving young people with such health conditions in physical activity, you can enable all pupils to engage in and achieve through safe, effective and enjoyable physical activity.

8

Health-Related Learning for 5- to 7-Year-Olds

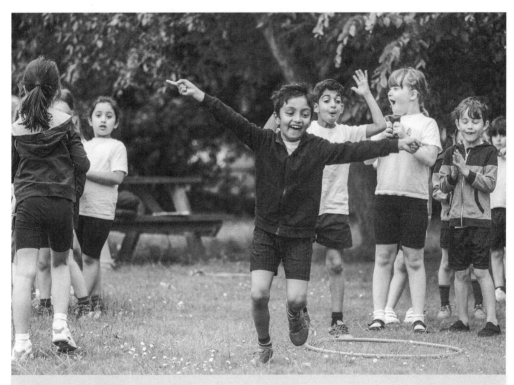

Chapter Objectives

After reading this chapter, you will be able to

- ▶ identify appropriate health-related learning outcomes and contexts for 5- to 7-year-olds;
- ▶ implement a variety of approaches to assess the health-related learning of 5- to 7-year-olds;
- ▶ describe methods for monitoring the health, activity and fitness of 5- to 7-year-olds; and
- ▶ create long-, medium- and short-term plans for health-related learning for 5- to 7-year-olds.

Children need to begin learning how to lead a healthy, active lifestyle at an early age, and this education should be formally structured and accessible to all pupils. The learning can be organised in multiple ways, including through PE lessons and focused topics. This chapter proposes health-related learning approaches for 5- to 7-year-olds and provides you with guidance for assessing this learning. It also suggests methods for monitoring the health, activity and fitness of 5- to 7-year-olds, such as simple health behaviour questionnaires, activity diaries and fitness-related activities. Finally, the chapter provides sample schemes, units of work and lesson plans to help you create health-related learning plans that ensure a comprehensive, coherent and meaningful approach to this important aspect of the curriculum.

Health-Related Learning Outcomes and Contexts

As detailed in chapter 3, approaches to health-related learning for the 5- to 16-year-old age group were debated and agreed on in England in 2000 by a working group comprising representatives of national PE, sport and health organisations. Table 8.1 presents specific health-related learn-ing outcomes for 5- to 7-year-olds; the outcomes are presented in four categories—safety issues, exercise effects, health benefits and activity pro-motion—to help clarify the scope and progression of the learning.

The learning content detailed in table 8.1 can be taught in a number of contexts. One approach is to integrate it into or permeate it through curriculum PE (e.g., during the teaching of dance, games and gymnastics lessons). Another approach, which is particularly appropriate for the 5- to 7-year-old age group as it aligns with the holistic approach to education often adopted in primary schools, is to teach health-related content in thematic or topic-based blocks or units of work with titles such as Healthy Me. A third option is to combine the first two approaches. Limitations in these approaches (discussed in chapter 3) can be addressed by ensuring that learning outcomes integrated into or permeated through curriculum PE are not lost and do not take second place to other learning (e.g., skill development). In addi-tion, in order to ensure consistency and coherence of health messages, learning outcomes taught in thematic or topic-based (or project-based) segments should be connected closely with the content and delivery of related subjects (e.g., PE; science; personal, social, health and economic [PSHE] education) and with relevant extracur-ricular and community activity experiences.

TABLE 8.1   Health-Related Learning Outcomes for Ages 5 to 7

Pupils who are 5 to 7 years old can do the following:

Safety issues	• Identify and adhere to safety rules and practices (e.g., changing clothes for PE lessons; tying long hair back; not wearing jewellery; sitting and standing with good posture; wearing footwear when skipping with a rope; not running fast to touch walls). • Explain that activity starts with a gentle warm-up and finishes with a calming cool-down.

Exercise effects	• Recognise, describe and feel the effects of exercise, including changes to
	  • breathing (e.g., it becomes faster and deeper),
	  • heart rate (e.g., heart pumps faster),
	  • temperature (e.g., person feels hotter),
	  • appearance (e.g., person looks hotter),
	  • feelings (e.g., person feels good, more energetic, tired) and
	  • external body parts (e.g., arm and leg muscles are working).
	• Explain that the body uses food and drink to release energy for exercise.

Health benefits	• Explain that regular exercise improves health by
	  • helping one feel good (e.g., happy, pleased, content) and
	  • helping body parts (e.g., bones, muscles) grow, develop and work well.

Activity promotion	• Identify when, where and how they can be active at school (both in and out of lessons). • Use opportunities to be active, including at playtimes.

More specifically, the learning outcomes related to safety issues can be taught in PE lessons and should be cross-referenced to related areas of the curriculum such as PSHE education, in which 5- to 7-year-olds are taught rules for and ways of staying physically and emotionally safe (PSHE Association, 2014). The outcomes related to exercise effects can be taught in PE lessons and cross-referenced to learning in related subjects such as science. The outcomes related to health benefits can be taught in PE lessons and are also relevant to elements of PSHE education (e.g., knowing what constitutes a healthy lifestyle) (PSHE Association, 2014) and therefore can be taught within thematic topics or projects (e.g., Healthy Me) with explicit links to learning in PE. And the outcomes related to activity promotion can be taught in PE lessons and also align with a whole-school approach to health (including the promotion of physical activity) and therefore can be taught within thematic topics or projects (e.g., Healthy Me) with explicit links to learning in PE. In keeping with a whole-school approach to health and physical activity promotion, information about activity opportunities on offer in the school and in the local community can be communicated to pupils and their families via newsletters, posters, parent mail, parent consultations, assemblies and the school website. For example, a Where to Be Active section can be cre-ated on the school website to advertise physical activity opportunities both at school and within a five-mile radius of the school; this section can also be used to connect and support pupils (and families) involved in these activities.

Assessing Health-Related Learning

Health-related learning can be assessed via written, spoken and active responses to questions, tasks and tests. In terms of focus, assessment can address affective, behavioural and cognitive (ABC) learning outcomes; for more on ABC outcomes, see chapter 3. Affective and behavioural outcomes for 5- to 7-year-olds can be assessed via teacher observation of effort and commitment in PE lessons, as well as participation records for PE lessons and extracurricular activities (using ratings such as excellent, good, satisfactory or adequate, and low or inadequate). Cognitive outcomes can be assessed through question-and-answer episodes and through practical and active tasks. Active assessment tasks are particularly encouraged because they increase activity levels in PE lessons (for more about active assessment, see chapter 3). Table 8.2 presents a range of methods for assessing the recommended health-related learning outcomes for 5- to 7-year-olds.

TABLE 8.2 Methods of Assessing Health-Related Learning in 5- to 7-Year-Olds

Health-related learning category	Health-related learning outcomes	Methods of assessing health-related learning outcomes

Safety issues	• Identify and adhere to safety rules and practices (e.g., changing clothes for PE lessons; tying long hair back; not wearing jewellery; sitting and standing with good posture; wearing footwear when skipping with a rope; not running fast to touch walls).
	• Explain that activity starts with a gentle warm-up and finishes with a calming cool-down.
		• Observe adherence to safety rules and practices.
		• Ask pupils questions, such as:
		  • Why do we change for PE?
		  • What rules help us keep safe in PE?
		  • What do we do at the beginning of a PE lesson to prepare for energetic activity?
		  • What do we do at the end of a PE lesson to recover from being energetic?
		• Involve pupils in active assessment tasks, such as:
		  • Show me how to sit with good posture (i.e., back tall, shoulders down, chest out, face forward).
		  • Demonstrate standing with good posture (i.e., feet apart, hips square, back tall, shoulders down, chest out, face forward).

(continued)

Table 8.2 *(continued)*

Health-related learning category	Health-related learning outcomes	Methods of assessing health-related learning outcomes

Exercise effects	• Recognise, describe and feel the effects of exercise, including changes to
	  • breathing (e.g., it becomes faster and deeper),
	  • heart rate (e.g., heart pumps faster),
	  • temperature (e.g., person feels hotter),
	  • appearance (e.g., person looks hotter),
	  • feelings (e.g., person feels good, more energetic, tired) and
	  • external body parts (e.g., arm and leg muscles are working).
	• Explain that the body uses food and drink to release energy for exercise.
		• Ask pupils questions, such as:
		  • What happens to your breathing when you exercise?
		  • What happens to your heart rate when you exercise?
		  • What happens to your body temperature when you exercise?
		  • How do you feel when you exercise?
		  • What happens to your body parts (e.g., arm and leg muscles) when you exercise?
		  • Where do you get energy to exercise?
		• Involve pupils in active assessment tasks, such as:
		  • Show me how you can make your heart pump faster.
		  • Show me some activities to make your breathing faster.
		  • Demonstrate activities that you enjoy doing.

Health benefits	• Explain that regular exercise improves health by
	  • helping one feel good (e.g., happy, pleased, content) and
	  • helping body parts (e.g., bones, muscles) grow, develop and work well.
		• Ask pupils questions, such as:
		  • How does being active help you be healthy?
		  • How do you feel when you exercise?
		  • Do you like being active by yourself?
		  • Do you like being active with others?
		  • How does exercise help parts of the body (e.g., bones, muscles) work well?
		• Involve pupils in active assessment tasks, such as:
		  • Show me an activity that helps you feel good.
		  • Demonstrate activities or exercises that help your bones and muscles become stronger.

Activity promotion	• Identify when, where and how they can be active at school (both in and out of lessons).
	• Use opportunities to be active, including at break times.
		• Observe informal activity (e.g., in the hall or on the playground) before and after school and during breaks and lunchtimes.
		• Record involvement in formal activities and clubs before, during and after school.
		• Have pupils pair up and tell their partners what activities they do at school, with whom, and what they think of each activity.
		• Ask pupils questions, such as:
		  • When and where can you be active on school days?
		  • Do you know how to join school activities?
		  • Who is active before school, during breaks, at lunchtimes and after school? Also, what do you do? Where and with whom?
		• Involve pupils in active assessment tasks, such as:
		  • Mime an activity that you can do at school; ask a partner to guess what the activity is.
		  • Show me a poster in the classroom (or school) about school activities or clubs.
		  • Demonstrate where to find information about school activities and clubs.

Monitoring Health, Activity and Fitness

The rationale for monitoring children's health, activity and fitness has been strengthened in recent years both by increased concern about children's physical, mental and social health and by the trend towards sedentary living that marks a more technologically advanced world. These issues are addressed in detail in part I of this book, whereas part II covers developmentally and pedagogically appropriate approaches to monitoring within the curriculum in order to promote healthy, active lifestyles among children. The following examples are appropriate for use with 5- to 7-year-olds.

Monitoring Health

We can help young children become more aware of their lifestyles by using health behaviour questionnaires (see chapter 4) that ask simple questions such as the following:

- Do you eat fruits and vegetables each day? Where do you do this?
- Do you drink water each day? Where do you do this?
- Are you active every day? Where do you do this?

Responses to these questions can trigger discussions about ways to become and remain healthy. When conducting such discussions, be sensitive to the fact that young children have no control over major factors that influence their health—for example, genetics, environment (e.g., pollution, poverty) and family modelling. In addition, they have only limited control over other key factors, including what they eat and drink and how active they are. So, whilst young children can learn about what constitutes a healthy lifestyle (as advocated in national curricula), they cannot be held responsible for—and should not be made to feel guilty about—the lifestyle they lead or their state of health. Furthermore, leading a healthy lifestyle can cost more in terms of purchasing healthy foods and drinks and accessing physical activity opportunities (e.g., after-school or holiday clubs) that require payment. As a consequence, young children from low-income families may be disadvantaged in comparison with their peers and, where possible, should be offered free or low-cost opportunities to consume healthy meals and drinks and to be active.

Monitoring Activity

As described in chapter 5, children's physical activity can be monitored through a number of methods. Appropriate methods for 5- to 7-year-olds include proxy reports (in which parents or teachers report children's activity via a simple form) and direct observation of children's activity (in which the type, intensity and duration of activity are recorded on a coding form or hand-held device). Direct observation is considered a particularly appropriate method for capturing the sporadic and transitory nature of young children's activity.

Whilst obtaining a precise measure of physical activity is important for research purposes, it is less crucial for teachers, whose main concerns relate to the educational value of the monitoring experience and its ease of use, feasibility and cost. From a pedagogical perspective, it is considered more important to ensure that pupils enjoy, learn and benefit from the monitoring experience than to focus unduly on the precision of the method (Cale & Harris, 2009b). This learning can include gaining insight into when, where and how they can be active in the school setting, which reflects the activity promotion outcomes for 5- to 7-year-olds shown in table 8.1.

Children's awareness of their physical activity levels can be increased by asking them to reflect on how active they are. For example, young pupils can be encouraged to talk, or write a short story, about what physical activity they do and where they do it; their responses can then be used to prompt discussion about healthy, active lifestyles. Another approach is to present young pupils with a predetermined list of activities (e.g., walking, cycling, skipping, tag or chase, ball games, swimming, dance, football) and ask them to tick those that they do and write or talk about where they do them. You can also incorporate questions about sedentary behaviour into discussions about healthy lifestyles. This approach links with the UK-wide physical activity guideline that children and young people should minimise the amount of time spent being sedentary (for more information about these guidelines, see chapter 1). Young children's responses to questions such as 'Do you sometimes sit down for a long time?' and 'Where do you sit down for a long time?' can be used to

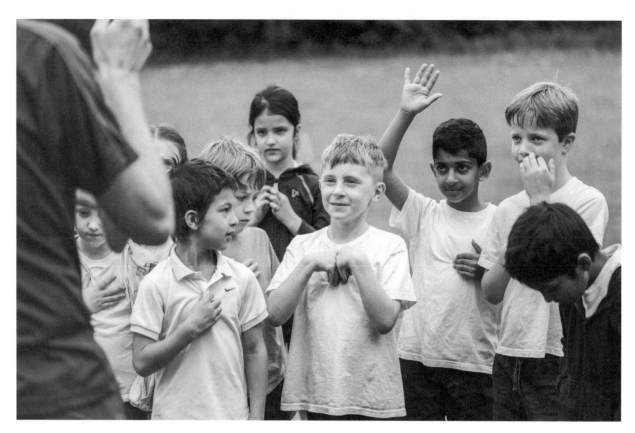

Primary school teachers can help young children to learn about the physical, mental and social health benefits of being active.

promote discussion about how it might be possible to fit more activity into the day.

Monitoring Fitness

As discussed in chapter 6, fitness testing is controversial in a school setting, and before using it with children we must consider a number of issues and limitations. Fitness monitoring can be considered a valuable component of the curriculum if it is developmentally appropriate; offers a positive, educational experience for all learners; and helps promote healthy, active lifestyles (Association for Physical Education [afPE], 2015; Cale, 2016; Cale & Harris, 2009a, 2009b; Cale, Harris, & Chen, 2014; Lloyd, Colley, & Tremblay, 2010; Rowland, 2007; Silverman, Keating, & Phillips, 2008). It is questionable, however, whether fitness tests are developmentally appropriate for children under the age of nine, given that many fitness tests require maximal effort to exhaustion and were designed for use with older children or adults. Indeed, the Association for Physical Education

(afPE; 2015) has published a position statement declaring that it does not support formal fitness testing in primary schools; moreover, it views such testing as a retrograde step in terms of promoting healthy, active lifestyles. The main reasons cited for this stance are that fitness testing does not necessarily constitute a good use of the limited curriculum time in primary schools; that it is not proven effective for promoting active lifestyles; that it can be dull, dreary and dreaded, especially by the very children whom we want to be more active; and that fitness test scores can be misleading and do not accurately reflect physical activity levels (afPE, 2015).

It is nevertheless useful to help young children understand that fitness is developed by being physically active. This understanding aligns with the goal of influencing the *process* (being active) rather than the *product* (fitness) (Cale & Harris, 2009b); it also reinforces the message that being active helps improve one's fitness and promotes good health. To facilitate such understanding, young pupils can be encouraged to write a short

FIVE A DAY

As part of a PhD study, a teacher in a state primary school in the Midlands investigated the effects of a physical activity intervention on the learning and physical activity behaviour of children aged 5 to 11. The intervention consisted of five minutes of physical activity every day for a school term (10 weeks), as well as delivery of associated health messages. It was facilitated by class teachers, who were involved in designing the intervention and contributed suggestions for activities that would be appealing, accessible and manageable. Ideas included walking, jogging, skipping and jumping; throwing, catching and kicking a ball; and playground games and movement to music. The health messages included the following: activity can help you be healthy, being active is fun, be active for an hour a day, some activity is better than none, everyone can be active, you don't need any particular skills, activity can help you feel good about yourself, and activity can help you make new friends. The intervention occurred within the curriculum and at a time and place each day that was considered appropriate by the class teachers.

Discussion points: What are the advantages of involving class teachers in designing the intervention? In what ways can activities be made accessible to all pupils?

The children's learning was measured by means of literacy and numeracy tests (which were conducted routinely in the school) and a questionnaire designed to assess children's knowledge and understanding of health, activity and fitness. The children's physical activity behaviour was monitored via physical activity diaries and accelerometer data (from a selected sample of pupils). In addition, the class teachers kept journals to record information related to the feasibility of the intervention and pupils' responses to it. Data from all of these sources were collected before and after the intervention, and comparisons were made between control and intervention classes.

Discussion points: What are your views on the methods used to measure the children's learning and physical activity behaviour? What are the pros and cons of an experimental research design involving control and intervention classes?

The findings suggested that the intervention succeeded in developing children's knowledge and understanding of health, activity and fitness and that it increased children's physical activity during the period of the intervention and for a short time afterwards. However, it had no significant effect (positive or negative) on children's literacy and numeracy. Teachers reported that the intervention was enthusiastically received in the first few weeks of the term but that some children's motivation fell off after this time, especially among the 9- to 11-year-olds, and it proved challenging to maintain their interest in the activities offered.

Discussion points: Are the findings what you expected them to be? What were the study's limitations? Could this type of intervention be implemented in other primary schools?

story or create a drawing about what fitness means to them and how they can become more active, more fit and healthier.

Health-Related Learning Plans for 5- to 7-Year-Olds

Long-term health-related plans generally take the form of a scheme of work over a number of years. In the case of 5- to 7-year-olds, the duration of the scheme of work is two academic years. Ideally, the health-related learning sits within a whole-school approach to the promotion of health, including physical activity (see chapter 2), and can be taught within a number of contexts—for example, integrating it into or permeating it through curriculum PE (e.g., teaching it through dance, games and gymnastics) and teaching it in thematic or topic-based blocks or units of work. Learning outcomes that are integrated into or permeated through curriculum PE should not be lost or allowed to take second place to other learning (e.g., skill development), and outcomes addressed through topics or projects should relate closely to the content and delivery of curriculum PE and related subjects (e.g., science).

Sample Health-Related Scheme of Work for 5- to 7-Year-Olds

The health-related learning identified in this example spans two academic years and is taught through a combination of curriculum PE and a topic-based project called Healthy Me. This learning sits within a whole-school approach to health that prioritises the promotion of physical activity, healthy eating and emotional well-being.

HEALTH-RELATED LEARNING CATEGORY: SAFETY ISSUES

HEALTH-RELATED LEARNING OUTCOMES

- Identify and adhere to safety rules and practices (e.g., changing clothes for PE lessons; tying long hair back; not wearing jewellery; sitting and standing with good posture; wearing footwear when skipping with a rope; not running fast to touch walls).
- Explain that activity starts with a gentle warm-up and finishes with a calming cool-down.

HEALTH-RELATED LEARNING CONTEXT

These learning outcomes are taught in PE lessons and cross-referenced to PSHE education in which pupils are taught rules for and ways of keeping physically and emotionally safe (PSHE Association, 2014).

METHODS OF ASSESSING HEALTH-RELATED LEARNING OUTCOMES

- Observe adherence to safety rules and practices.
- Ask pupils questions such as the following:
  - Why do we change for PE?
  - What rules help us keep safe in PE?
  - What do we do at the beginning of a PE lesson to prepare for energetic activity?
  - What do we do at the end of a PE lesson to recover from being energetic?
- Involve pupils in active assessment tasks such as the following:
  - Show me how to sit with good posture (back tall, shoulders down, chest out, face forward).
  - Demonstrate standing with good posture (feet apart, hips square, back tall, shoulders down, chest out, face forward).

HEALTH-RELATED LEARNING CATEGORY: EXERCISE EFFECTS

HEALTH-RELATED LEARNING OUTCOMES

- Recognise, describe and feel the effects of activity, including changes to
  - breathing (e.g., it becomes faster and deeper),
  - heart rate (e.g., heart pumps faster),
  - temperature (e.g., person feels hotter),
  - appearance (e.g., person looks hotter),
  - feelings (e.g., person feels good, more energetic, tired) and
  - external body parts (e.g., arm and leg muscles are working).
- Explain that the body uses food and drink to release energy for activity.

HEALTH-RELATED LEARNING CONTEXT

These learning outcomes are taught in PE lessons and cross-referenced to learning in science.

METHODS OF ASSESSING HEALTH-RELATED LEARNING OUTCOMES

- Ask pupils questions such as the following:
  - What happens to your breathing when you exercise?
  - What happens to your heart rate when you exercise?
  - What happens to your body temperature when you exercise?
  - How do you feel when you exercise?

- What happens to your body parts (e.g., arm and leg muscles) when you exercise?
- Where do you get energy to exercise?
- Involve pupils in active assessment tasks such as the following:

- Show me how you can make your heart pump faster.
- Show me some activities to make your breathing faster.
- Demonstrate activities that you enjoy doing.

HEALTH-RELATED LEARNING CATEGORY: HEALTH BENEFITS

HEALTH-RELATED LEARNING OUTCOMES

Explain that regular activity improves health by

- helping one feel good (e.g., happy, pleased, content) and
- helping body parts (e.g., bones, muscles) grow, develop and work well.

HEALTH-RELATED LEARNING CONTEXT

These learning outcomes are addressed within the Healthy Me project that covers related PSHE education content (e.g., knowing what constitutes a healthy lifestyle) (PSHE Association, 2014) and are cross-referenced to learning in PE.

METHODS OF ASSESSING HEALTH-RELATED LEARNING OUTCOMES

- Ask pupils questions such as the following:
  - How does being active help you to be healthy?
  - How do you feel when you exercise?
  - Do you like being active by yourself?
  - Do you like being active with others?
  - How does exercise help parts of the body (e.g., bones, muscles) work well?
- Involve pupils in active assessment tasks such as the following:
  - Show me an activity that helps you feel good.
  - Demonstrate activities or exercises that help your bones and muscles become stronger.

HEALTH-RELATED LEARNING CATEGORY: ACTIVITY PROMOTION

HEALTH-RELATED LEARNING OUTCOMES

- Identify when, where and how they can be active at school (both in and out of lessons).
- Use opportunities to be active, including at break times.

HEALTH-RELATED LEARNING CONTEXT

These learning outcomes are addressed within the Healthy Me project and cross-referenced to learning in PE. In particular, they align with a whole-school approach to health, including the promotion of physical activity. Information about activity opportunities on offer in the school and in the local community is communicated to pupils and their families via newsletters, posters, parent mail, parent consultations, assemblies and the school website.

METHODS OF ASSESSING HEALTH-RELATED LEARNING OUTCOMES

- Observe informal activity (e.g., in the hall or playground) before and after school and during breaks and lunchtimes.
- Record involvement in formal activities and clubs before, during and after school.
- Have pupils pair up and tell their partners what activities they do at school, with whom, and what they think of them.
- Ask pupils questions such as the following:
  - When and where can you be active on school days?
  - Do you know how to join school activities?

– Who is active before school, during breaks, at lunchtimes and after school? What do you do? Where, and with whom?

- Involve pupils in active assessment tasks such as the following:

  – Mime an activity that you can do at school; ask a partner to guess what the activity is.

– Show me a poster in the classroom (or school) about school activities or clubs.

– Demonstrate where to find information about school activities and clubs.

Medium-term plans for health-related learning generally take the form of units or blocks of work that last for a school term (usually 10 to 14 weekly lessons) or part of a term (usually 4 to 7 weekly lessons). This learning is likely to be situated within the subject of PE or in thematic or topic-based (or project-based) units or blocks of work.

Sample Health-Related Unit of Work for 5- to 7-Year-Olds

The following example presents a four-lesson, topic-based unit called Healthy Me and outlines selected learning outcomes for health benefits and activity promotion for 6- and 7-year-olds. It also covers learning activities to address the outcomes, as well as suggested methods for assessing pupils' learning. The learning in this unit is cross-referenced to related learning in PE.

HEALTH-RELATED LEARNING OUTCOMES: LESSONS 1 AND 2

HEALTH BENEFITS

- Explain that regular activity improves health by
  - helping you feel good (e.g., happy, pleased, content) and
  - helping body parts (e.g., bones, muscles) grow, develop and work well.

HEALTH-RELATED LEARNING ACTIVITIES

- Ask: What do you think *health* means?

  Encourage pupils to think about physical, mental and social health—that is, body and mind working well, feeling happy or good and enjoying time with family and friends.

- Ask: What can you do to be healthy?

  Encourage pupils to think about a range of behaviours associated with good physical, mental and social health. Examples include being active, eating and drinking healthy foods and drinks, getting a good night's sleep, having fun and playing with family and friends.

- Ask: How does being active help you be healthy?

  Encourage pupils to think about a range of physical, mental and social benefits—for example, feeling good, enjoying playing with friends, having a healthy and efficient heart and strong arm and leg muscles.

- Over two lessons, involve pupils in a range of simple whole-body activities, such as walking, jogging, moving to music, skipping, hopping and galloping.

  In the second lesson, arrange for some of these activities to be done with peers and encourage social interaction (e.g., chatting whilst walking, skipping with a long rope in small groups).

- Afterwards, ask: Which activities did you like best? What did you like about them? Did you enjoy the activities you did by yourself? What did you enjoy or not enjoy about it? Did you enjoy the activities you did with others? What did you enjoy or not enjoy about it?

ASSESSMENT OF HEALTH-RELATED LEARNING

- Towards the end of the unit of work, ask pupils questions such as the following:
  - How does being active help you be healthy?
  - How do you feel when you exercise?
  - Do you like being active by yourself?
  - Do you like being active with others?
  - How does exercise help parts of the body (e.g., bones, muscles) work well?

- Towards the end of the unit of work, involve pupils in active assessment tasks such as the following:
  - Show me an activity that helps you feel good.
  - Demonstrate activities or exercises that help your bones and muscles become stronger.

HEALTH-RELATED LEARNING OUTCOMES: LESSONS 3 AND 4

ACTIVITY PROMOTION

- Identify when, where and how they can be active at school (both in and out of lessons).
- Use opportunities to be active, including at break times.

HEALTH-RELATED LEARNING ACTIVITIES

- Ask: Where and when can you be active at school?

  Encourage pupils to think about informal activity opportunities (e.g., in the hall or playground) before and after school; during breaks and lunchtimes; and during PE lessons and activities and clubs before, during and after school. Also prompt pupils to consider active travel to and from school, such as walking or scooting.

- Ask: How can you join in with these activities?

  Encourage pupils who are involved in before-school, lunchtime and after-school clubs to talk about how they joined and how it felt to do so. Also, discuss ways of joining in with informal activity opportunities in the hall or playground at various times of the school day.

- Ask: Which activities do you already join in with?

  Provide prompts about active travel to school, informal play, PE lessons and formal clubs and activities.

- Over two lessons, involve pupils in a selection of activities available at school, including playground games such as tag and hopscotch.

  In the second of the two lessons, encourage pupils to make up their own games and activities by using markings on the ground or walls (e.g., lines, circles, targets) and simple equipment such as cones and markers.

- Afterwards, ask: Which playground activities did you like best? What did you like about them? Did you enjoy making up your own activities or games? Was there anything that you did not enjoy about it? What could have made it more enjoyable?

ASSESSMENT OF HEALTH-RELATED LEARNING

- Towards the end of the unit of work, ask pupils questions such as the following:
  - When and where can you be active on school days?
  - Do you know how to join school activities?
  - Who is active before school, during breaks, at lunchtimes and after school? What do you do? Where, and with whom?

- Also have pupils pair up and tell their partners what activities they do at school, with whom, and what they think of them.

- Where possible during the unit of work, do the following:
  - Observe the pupils' informal activity (e.g., in the hall or playground) before and after school and during breaks and lunchtimes.
  - Record pupils' involvement in formal activities and clubs before, during and after school.

- Towards the end of the unit of work, involve pupils in active assessment tasks such as the following:
  - Mime an activity that you can do at school; ask a partner to guess what the activity is.

- Show me a poster in the classroom (or school) about school activities and clubs.
- Demonstrate where to find information about school activities and clubs.

Short-term plans for health-related learning generally take the form of lesson plans with specific health-related learning outcomes that sit within units or blocks of work. The following example is a lesson plan for 5- to 6-year-olds that outlines selected learning activities for exercise effects, as well as learning activities to address the outcomes and suggested methods of assessing the learning.

HEALTH-RELATED LEARNING OUTCOMES

EXERCISE EFFECTS

- Recognise, describe and feel the effects of activity, including changes to
  - breathing (e.g., it becomes faster and deeper),
  - heart rate (e.g., heart pumps faster),
  - temperature (e.g., person feels hotter),
  - appearance (e.g., person looks hotter) and
  - feelings (e.g., person feels good, more energetic, tired).

HEALTH-RELATED LEARNING ACTIVITIES

- Starting in the centre of the learning area (either indoors or outdoors), ask pupils to put a hand on their chest to feel their breathing. Ask: How would you describe your breathing at the moment? (Sample answers: gentle, slow.) What do you think will happen to your breathing after we do some activity? (Become faster, quicker, harder.)
- Ask pupils to walk to touch all four corners of the area, in any order, while being careful not to walk into other people.
- When they return to the centre, ask: How would you describe your breathing now? (Faster, quicker, harder.) How do you feel? (Okay, a little out of breath, warm.)
- Put your hand over your heart to feel it working. Can you feel a pulse? How hard is your heart working at the moment? (Slowly, not

very hard.) What do you think will happen to your heart rate after we do some energetic activity? (Become faster, quicker, harder.)
- Ask pupils to *jog* to touch all four corners of the area, in any order, while being careful not to jog into other people.
- When they return to the centre, ask pupils to put a hand over their heart again. Ask: How hard is your heart working now? (Faster, quicker, harder.) How do you feel now? (Tired, out of breath, hot.)
- Ask pupils to run on the spot, starting slowly and getting gradually faster (going up from first gear to fifth gear).
- Afterwards, ask pupils to put a hand over their heart again. Ask: How hard is your heart working now? (Much faster, quicker, or harder.) How do you feel now? (Tired, good, very hot, sweaty.)
- Ask pupils to show you an activity that makes their heart work steadily (not fast and not slow). Then ask them to demonstrate an activity that makes their breathing slow.
- Afterwards, prompt: Describe your breathing (slow, calm). Describe your heart rate (slow, calm, quiet). How do you feel now? (OK, good, relaxed, calm, a little tired.)

ASSESSMENT OF HEALTH-RELATED LEARNING

- What happens to your breathing when you exercise?

- What happens to your heart rate when you exercise?
- What happens to your body temperature when you exercise?
- What happens to your body parts (e.g., arm and leg muscles) when you exercise?
- Show me how you can make your heart pump faster (or slower).
- Show me some activities you can do to make your breathing faster (or slower).
- How do you feel when you exercise (or after you have exercised)?

An assessment form associated with this lesson is provided in the web resource for this chapter.

What Happens to Us When We Exercise?

What happens to your breathing when you exercise?	
What happens to your heart rate when you exercise?	
What happens to your body temperature when you exercise?	
What happens to your body parts (e.g., arm and leg muscles) when you exercise?	
How do you feel when you exercise?	

Show me how you can make your heart pump faster.

Show me some activities you can do to make your breathing faster.

Now, do some activities that make your heart pump slower.

How do you feel after you have exercised?

1   From J. Harris and L. Cale, 2018, *Promoting active lifestyles in schools web resource.* (Champaign, IL: Human Kinetics)

Summary

If you take a structured, progressive approach to children's learning about leading a healthy, active lifestyle, then you can engage pupils with this important aspect of the curriculum in a way that is comprehensive, coherent and meaningful. This sort of approach needs to be evident at all stages of schooling and be accessible to every pupil. A good way to start is to develop health-related learning plans that include relevant outcomes for successive age groups. The learning can then be organised, taught and assessed in multiple ways and can incorporate the monitoring of children's health, activity and fitness through methods that are developmentally appropriate and pedagogically desirable.

Health-Related Learning for 7- to 11-Year-Olds

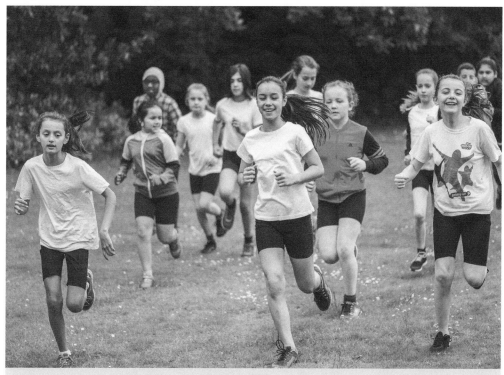

Chapter Objectives

After reading this chapter, you will be able to

- ▶ identify appropriate health-related learning outcomes and contexts for 7- to 11-year-olds;
- ▶ implement a variety of approaches to assess the health-related learning of 7- to 11-year-olds;
- ▶ describe methods for monitoring the health, activity and fitness of 7- to 11-year-olds; and
- ▶ create long-, medium- and short-term plans for health-related learning for 7- to 11-year-olds.

Children's learning about leading a healthy, active lifestyle should be formally structured, progressive and accessible to all pupils. The learning can be organised in multiple ways, including through PE lessons and focused topics. This chapter proposes health-related learning approaches for 7- to 11-year-olds and provides you with guidance for assessing this learning. It also suggests methods for monitoring the health, activity and fitness of 7- to 11-year-olds, such as health behaviour questionnaires, activity diaries and developmentally appropriate fitness tests and fitness-related activities. Finally, the chapter provides sample schemes, units of work and lesson plans to help you create health-related learning plans that ensure a comprehensive, coherent and meaningful approach to this important aspect of the curriculum.

Health-Related Learning Outcomes and Contexts

As detailed in chapter 3, approaches to health-related learning for the 5- to 16-year-old age group were debated and agreed on in England in 2000 by a working group comprising representatives of national PE, sport and health organisations. Table 9.1 presents specific health-related learning outcomes for 7- to 11-year-olds; the outcomes are presented in four categories—safety issues, exercise effects, health benefits and activity promotion—to help clarify the scope and progression of the learning.

The learning content detailed in table 9.1 can be taught in a number of contexts. One approach is to integrate it into or permeate it through curriculum PE (e.g., during the teaching of athletics, dance, games, gymnastics, outdoor education and swimming lessons). Another approach is to teach health-related content in thematic or topic-based blocks or units of work with titles such as Be Healthy and Active. A third option is to combine the first two approaches. Limitations in these approaches (discussed in chapter 3) can be addressed by ensuring that learning outcomes integrated into or permeated through curriculum PE are not lost and do not take second place to other learning (e.g., skill development, tactical understanding). In addition, in order to ensure consistency and coherence of health messages, learning outcomes taught in thematic or topic-based (or project-based) segments should be connected closely with the content and delivery of related subjects (e.g., PE; science; personal, social, health and economic [PSHE] education) and with extracurricular and community activity experiences.

More specifically, the learning outcomes related to safety issues can be taught in PE lessons and should be cross-referenced to related areas of the curriculum such as PSHE education, in which 7- to 11-year-olds are taught about keeping themselves and others safe (e.g., protecting themselves from dehydration and sunburn) (PSHE Association, 2014). The outcomes related to exercise effects can be taught in PE lessons and also lend themselves to cross-curricular links with related subjects such as science. The outcomes related to health benefits can be taught in PE lessons and are also relevant to PSHE education (e.g., learning to make informed choices and beginning to understand the concept of a balanced lifestyle) (PSHE Association, 2014) and therefore can be taught within thematic topics or projects (e.g., Be Healthy and Active) with explicit links to learning in PE. And the outcomes related to activity promotion can be taught in PE lessons and also align with a whole-school approach to health (including the promotion of physical activity) and therefore can be taught within thematic topics or projects (e.g., Be Healthy and Active) with explicit links to learning in PE.

In keeping with a whole-school approach to health and physical activity promotion, information about activity opportunities on offer in the school and in the local community can be communicated to pupils and their families via newsletters, posters, parent mail, parent consultations, assemblies and the school website. For example, a Where to Be Active section can be created on the school website to advertise physical activity opportunities both at school and within a five-mile radius of the school; this section can also be used to connect and support pupils (and families) involved in these activities.

Assessing Health-Related Learning

Health-related learning can be assessed via written, verbal and active responses to questions, tasks and tests. In terms of focus, assessment can address affective, behavioural and cognitive (ABC) learning outcomes; for more on ABC outcomes,

TABLE 9.1 Health-Related Learning Outcomes for Ages 7 to 11

Pupils who are 7 to 11 years old can do the following:

Safety issues	• Explain the need for safety rules and practices (e.g., adopting good posture at all times; being hygienic; changing clothes and having a wash after energetic activity; wearing footwear as appropriate; following rules; protecting against cold weather; avoiding sunburn; lifting safely; using space sensibly [not bumping into others]). • Identify the purpose of warming up and of cooling down and recognise and describe the parts of a warm-up and of a cool-down: exercises for the joints (e.g., arm circles), whole-body activities (e.g., jogging, skipping without a rope) and stretches for either the whole body (e.g., reaching long and tall) or parts of the body (e.g., lower-leg or calf muscles).

Exercise effects	• Explain and feel the short-term effects of exercise:
	  • Breathing rate and depth increase to provide more oxygen to working muscles.
	  • Heart rate increases to pump more oxygen to working muscles.
	  • Temperature increases because working muscles produce energy in the form of heat; as that heat is transferred to the body's surface (skin) to control body temperature, the skin can become moist, sticky and sweaty.
	  • Appearance can become flushed due to blood vessels widening and getting closer to the surface of the skin.
	  • Feelings and moods can vary (e.g., having fun, feeling good among friends).
	• Explain that the body needs a certain amount of energy every day in the form of food and drink in order to function properly (e.g., for normal growth, development and daily living) and that body fat increases if more calories are taken in than are needed (e.g., for breathing, growing, sleeping, eating, moving, exercise).

Health benefits	• Explain that activity strengthens bones and muscles (including the heart) and helps keep joints flexible. • Explain that activity can help one feel good about oneself and can be fun and social (e.g., involves sharing experiences and cooperating with others). • Explain that regular activity enables one to perform daily activities more easily. • Explain that being active helps one maintain a healthy body weight.
Activity promotion	• Monitor their current levels of activity (e.g., daily, twice weekly). • Identify when, where and how they can be active, both in school and outside of school. • Make decisions about which physical activities they enjoy and explain that individuals have different feelings about the types and amounts of activity they do. • Use opportunities to be active for 30 to 60 minutes a day (with rest periods as necessary), including lessons, playtimes and club activities.

see chapter 3. Affective and behavioural outcomes for 7- to 11-year-olds can be assessed via teacher observation of effort and commitment in PE lessons, as well as participation records for PE lessons and extracurricular activities (using ratings such as excellent, good, satisfactory or adequate, and low or inadequate). Cognitive outcomes can be assessed through question-and-answer episodes and through practical and active tasks. Active assessment tasks are particularly encouraged because they increase activity levels in PE lessons (for more information about active assessment, see chapter 3). Table 9.2 presents a range of methods for assessing the recommended health-related learning outcomes for 7- to 11-year-olds.

Monitoring Health, Activity and Fitness

The rationale for monitoring children's health, activity and fitness has been strengthened in recent years both by increased concern about children's physical, mental and social health and by the trend towards sedentary living that marks a more technologically advanced world. These issues are addressed in part I of this book, whereas part II covers developmentally and pedagogically appropriate approaches to monitoring within the curriculum in order to promote healthy, active lifestyles among children.

TABLE 9.2 Methods of Assessing Health-Related Learning in 7- to 11-Year-Olds

Health-related learning category	Health-related learning outcomes	Methods of assessing health-related learning outcomes
Safety issues	• Explain the need for safety rules and practices (e.g., adopting good posture at all times; being hygienic; changing clothes and having a wash after energetic activity; wearing footwear as appropriate; following rules; protecting against cold weather; avoiding sunburn; lifting safely; using space sensibly [not bumping into others]). • Identify the purpose of warming up and of cooling down and recognise and describe the parts of a warm-up and of a cool-down: exercises for the joints (e.g., arm circles), whole-body activities (e.g., jogging, skipping without a rope) and stretches for either the whole body (e.g., reaching long and tall) or parts of the body (e.g., lower-leg or calf muscles).	• Ask pupils questions such as: • Why is good posture important? • Why do we change for activity? • Why do we wash after energetic activity? • Why is it sensible to wear trainers for activities such as jumping and playing games? • Discuss with a partner some rules in PE and sport. Why do we have rules? • Talk with a partner about how to avoid feeling cold in the winter. • Talk with a partner about how to avoid getting sunburnt. • Why do we warm up? • What is a cool-down, and what is it for? • Talk with a partner about the types of exercises included in a warm-up (or cool-down)? • Involve pupils in active assessment tasks such as: • Show me how to walk with good posture. • Demonstrate how to lift something heavy. • Show me some activities to warm up your whole body. • Show me an exercise for your shoulders (or hips). • Demonstrate a whole-body stretch.
Exercise effects	• Explain and feel the short-term effects of exercise: • Breathing rate and depth increase to provide more oxygen to working muscles. • Heart rate increases to pump more oxygen to working muscles. • Temperature increases because working muscles produce energy in the form of heat; as that heat is transferred to the body's surface (skin) to control body temperature, the skin can become moist, sticky and sweaty. • Appearance can become flushed due to blood vessels widening and getting closer to the surface of the skin. • Feelings and moods can vary (e.g., having fun, feeling friendly). • Explain that the body needs a certain amount of energy every day in the form of food and drink in order to function properly (e.g., for normal growth, development and daily living) and that body fat increases if more calories are taken in than are needed (e.g., for breathing, growing, sleeping, eating, moving, exercise).	• Ask pupils questions such as: • How does your breathing change when you are active? • Why does it do this? • Why does your heart rate change when you are active? • What happens to your body temperature when you are active, and why? • Why do we sometimes sweat when we are active? • Talk with a partner about why our appearance can change when we do energetic activity. • How do you feel when you are active (e.g., jogging, dancing, playing games)? • What does the body need energy for? Where does this energy come from? • How much food and drink does the body need? • What can happen if the body has too much (or too little) food and drink? • Involve pupils in active assessment tasks such as: • Show me how you can increase your heart rate and breathing rate. • Demonstrate some activities that make you warm (or hot).

Health-related learning category	Health-related learning outcomes	Methods of assessing health-related learning outcomes

Health benefits	• Explain that activity strengthens bones and muscles (including the heart) and helps keep joints flexible.
	• Explain that activity can help one feel good about oneself and can be fun and social (e.g., sharing experiences and cooperating with others).
	• Explain that regular activity permits one to perform daily activities more easily.
	• Explain that being active helps one maintain a healthy body weight.
		• Ask pupils questions such as:
		  • How does being active strengthen bones and muscles?
		  • How can being active help you in everyday life?
		  • How does activity help you achieve and maintain a healthy weight?
		  • Talk with a partner about activities that you like, how they make you feel, and why you like them.
		  • Name some activities in which you must work together to do well.
		• Involve pupils in active assessment tasks such as:
		  • Show me an activity that strengthens bones and muscles.
		  • Demonstrate exercises that help keep your joints flexible.

Activity promotion	• Monitor their current levels of activity (e.g., daily, twice weekly).
	• Identify when, where and how they can be active, both in school and outside of school.
	• Make decisions about which physical activities they enjoy and explain that individuals have different feelings about the types and amounts of activity they do.
	• Use opportunities to be active for 30 to 60 minutes a day (with rest periods as necessary), including lessons, playtimes and club activities.
		• Observe informal activity before and after school and during breaks and lunchtimes.
		• Record involvement in formal activities and clubs before, during and after school.
		• Have pupils keep an activity diary for one school day and one weekend day (recording all activity both at school and outside of school).
		• Have pupils show a partner their activity diary and discuss how much activity they did each day, where they did it, and with whom. Ask: Were you active for an hour per day on these days?
		• Discuss how to fit an hour of activity into a day. Ask questions such as:
		  • When and where can you be active, both in school and outside of school?
		• Talk with a partner about which activities you enjoy and which are your favourites. Are there any activities that you do not like so much? If so, what are they, and what do you not like about them?
		• Involve pupils in active assessment tasks such as:
		  • Show me where I can find out about activities outside of school.
		  • Mime one of your favourite activities (without equipment).
		  • Form a circle and take turns miming your favourite activities; after each mime, everyone copies it.

The following examples are appropriate for use with 7- to 11-year-olds.

Monitoring Health

We can help children become more aware of their lifestyles by using health behaviour questionnaires that offer a selection of responses (e.g., always, sometimes, never) to questions such as the following:

- Do you eat fruits and vegetables every day?
- Do you drink water every day?
- Are you active for about an hour every day?

The web resource for chapter 4 provides an example of a health behaviour questionnaire suitable for primary-age pupils; it can be used to calculate a health score linked to generic feedback such as the following: 'Well done, you lead a healthy lifestyle much of the time and will benefit from doing so. You might consider whether you could lead an even healthier lifestyle by adjusting some of your habits'. Engaging children in the process of self-reflection enhances learning and helps children to set measurable targets for improvement. Here is a sample question to ask of 7- to 11-year-olds: 'What parts of your health have you done well on? State one action that you can do to improve your health'. Additional examples of self-reflection questions are provided in chapter 4.

Responses to these questions can be used to trigger discussions among pupils about ways to lead a healthy lifestyle. When conducting such discussions, be sensitive to the fact that primary-age children have no control over major factors that influence their health—for example, genetics, environment (e.g., pollution, poverty) and family modelling. In addition, they have only limited control over other key factors, including what they eat and drink and how active they are. So, whilst children can learn about what constitutes a healthy lifestyle (as advocated in national curricula), they cannot be held responsible for—and should not be made to feel guilty about—the lifestyle they lead or their state of health. Furthermore, leading a healthy lifestyle can cost more in terms of purchasing healthy foods and drinks and accessing physical activity opportunities (e.g., after-school or holiday clubs) that require payment. As a consequence, children from low-income families may be disadvantaged in comparison with their peers and, where possible, should be offered free or low-cost opportunities to consume healthy meals and drinks and to be active.

Monitoring Activity

As described in chapter 5, children's physical activity can be monitored through a number of methods. Appropriate methods for 7- to 11-year-olds include proxy reports (in which parents or teachers report children's activity via a simple form) and direct observation of children's activity (in which the type, intensity and duration of activity are recorded on a coding form or handheld device). Pupils aged 7 to 11 years can also be asked to keep a physical activity diary for a school day and a weekend day (for examples of activity diaries suitable for this age group, see the web resource for chapter 5).

You can encourage pupils to reflect on their activity levels by asking questions such as the following: How active are you? Do you do enough physical activity for your age? What can you do to be more active? (For more examples appropriate for upper-primary-age children, see the web resource for chapter 5.)

You may also want to incorporate questions about sedentary behaviour into discussions about healthy lifestyles. This approach links with the UK-wide physical activity guideline that children and young people should minimise the amount of time spent being sedentary (for more information about these guidelines, see chapter 1). Young people's responses to questions such as 'Are there times when you sit down for a long time?', 'Are there places where you sit down for a long time?' and 'Could you be more active during these times or in these places?' can be used to promote discussion about inactivity and its consequences.

Whilst obtaining a precise measure of physical activity is important for research purposes, it is less crucial for teachers, whose main concerns relate to the educational value of the monitoring experience and its ease of use, feasibility and cost. From a pedagogical perspective, it is considered more important to ensure that pupils enjoy, learn and benefit from the monitoring experience than to focus unduly on the precision of the method (Cale & Harris, 2009b). This learning can include identifying when, where and how they can be active (including outside of school) and deciding which physical activities they enjoy (with the understanding that individuals have different preferences and feelings about types and amounts of activity).

Pupils should be encouraged to think of ways in which they could be more physically active, both in school and outside of school, and their responses can be used to prompt discussion about healthy, active lifestyles. Another approach is to ask pupils to tick the activities they do from a predetermined list (e.g., walking, cycling, skipping, tag or chase, ball games, swimming, dance, football) and state where they do them. Their responses can be shared with the class to increase awareness of activity opportunities in and beyond the school setting. Pupils can also be encouraged to draw, or create a poster about, what the word *activity* means to them and describe their creation to other pupils. You can use these visual images and descriptions to address any misunderstandings and misconceptions that children have about physical activity—for example, believing that it is only about sport and that activity must feel hard in order to be beneficial (see chapter 1 for a discussion of young people's inaccurate and inadequate understandings of health, fitness and physical activity).

Monitoring Fitness

As discussed in chapter 6, fitness testing is controversial in a school setting, and before using it with children we must consider a number of issues and limitations. Fitness monitoring can be considered a valuable component of the curriculum if it is developmentally appropriate; offers a positive, educational experience for all learners; and helps promote healthy, active lifestyles (Association for Physical Education [afPE], 2015; Cale, 2016; Cale & Harris, 2009a, 2009b; Cale, Harris, & Chen, 2014; Lloyd, Colley, & Tremblay, 2010; Rowland, 2007; Silverman, Keating, & Phillips, 2008). It is questionable, however, whether fitness tests are developmentally appropriate for children under the age of nine, given that many fitness tests

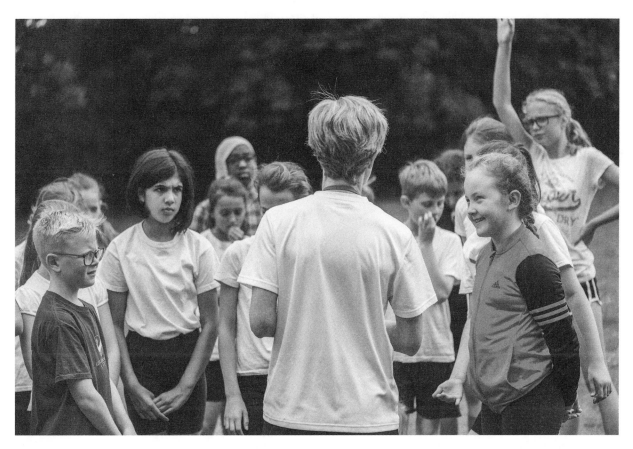

Teachers can help older primary school children to learn about the physical, mental and social health benefits of being active.

require maximal effort to exhaustion and were designed for use with older children or adults.

Indeed, the Association for Physical Education (afPE; 2015) has published a position statement declaring that it does not support formal fitness testing in primary schools; moreover, it views such testing as a retrograde step in terms of promoting healthy, active lifestyles. The main reasons for this stance are that fitness testing does not necessarily constitute a good use of the limited curriculum time in primary schools; that it is not proven effective for promoting active lifestyles; that it can be dull, dreary and dreaded,

especially by the very children whom we want to be more active; and that fitness test scores can be misleading and do not accurately reflect physical activity levels (afPE, 2015).

It is not essential for children aged 9 to 11 to be involved in formal fitness testing in order for them to learn that certain activities develop fitness (e.g., jogging and running improve cardiorespiratory fitness, and stretching improves flexibility). These associations can be taught in PE lessons, where children can learn, for example, that dance and gymnastics help develop their muscular strength and endurance and

A CROSS-CURRICULAR APPROACH TO ADOPTING AN ACTIVE WAY OF LIFE

Teachers in a primary school worked collectively to ensure strong cross-curricular links within a topic-based curriculum. One of the topics, Be Healthy and Active, was designed to address personal, social and health outcomes, particularly the adoption of an active way of life. The topic was developed by teachers responsible for physical education and science, as well as a member of the senior management team who had overall responsibility for the school's personal, social, health and economic education programme.

At the start of the topic, pupils completed an online questionnaire requiring them to list the health benefits of being active and identify activities they could do at school or in the local area (e.g., active travel to and from school; recreational and organised activities). Teachers used the questionnaire data to trigger discussions with pupils about the benefits of an active lifestyle over a sedentary one and about what helps children be active and what prevents them from doing so (e.g., not knowing where to be active, not having friends involved, not being able to afford it).

Discussion points: What uses could be made of the questionnaire data? How is it useful to find out why some pupils are not active?

Pupils were then asked to keep an activity diary for one school day and one weekend day. Afterward, they discussed their diary entries and were guided to consider whether they were meeting the 'one hour a day' activity recommendation and, if not, how they could be more active. Pupils were also asked to take a leaflet home to their parents outlining the health benefits of activity, providing information about the 'one hour a day' recommendation for children, and encouraging parents to promote activity as part of a healthy lifestyle. The leaflet also guided parents to the school website, which listed activities on offer at school and in the local leisure centre and sport clubs. It also informed parents about fun family events organised by the school involving activity (e.g., treasure hunt, Winter Waddle and Summer Stroll in the school grounds or a local park).

Discussion points: In what ways can schools provide pupils and parents with information about activity opportunities in the local community? What are your views on the communication to parents described in this case study?

In an annual review of the curriculum, the school concluded that the Be Healthy and Active topic was well received by pupils and resulted in an overall increase in health and activity knowledge and activity levels. It also provided a good opportunity to communicate important health messages to parents and support them in promoting healthy, active lifestyles with their children.

Discussion points: What are some ways in which this topic might be enhanced? What further support might schools provide to parents to help them promote healthy, active lifestyles?

also their flexibility (or, overall, their 'muscle health') and that games and running activities can improve their cardiorespiratory fitness (or 'heart health').

If you choose to involve 9- to 11-year-olds in formal fitness testing, select the tests carefully and teach them in a positive, supportive setting. Emphasise helping pupils enjoy and learn from the experience and strive to improve on their own personal-best scores. Submaximal tests are advised for this age group—for example, the step test and the mini bleep test for cardiorespiratory fitness and differentiated versions of exercises for muscular strength and endurance (e.g., curl-up, push-up). The chapter 6 web resource provides descriptions of these tests, as well as recommendations to consider before, during and after implementing them. Once fitness testing is completed, ask pupils to reflect on the experience and on their scores. The web resource for chapter 5 provides examples of appropriate questions for upper-primary-age children, such as the following: How did you feel about the tests? What do your scores tell you? What could you do to be more fit?

All children aged 7 to 11 years should be helped to understand that fitness is developed by being physically active and is associated with good health. This message is consistent with the goal of influencing the process (being active) rather than the product (fitness) (Cale & Harris, 2009b). In addition, pupils can be encouraged to draw, or create a poster about, what *fitness* means to them and to describe their creation to other pupils. You can use these visual images and descriptions to address any misunderstandings and misconceptions that children may have about fitness—for example, believing that it is about looking good and being thin (see chapter 1 for a discussion of young people's inaccurate and inadequate understandings of health, fitness and physical activity).

Health-Related Learning Plans for 7- to 11-Year-Olds

Long-term health-related plans generally take the form of a scheme of work over a number of years. In the case of 7- to 11-year-olds, the duration of the scheme of work is four academic years. Ideally, the health-related learning should sit within a whole-school approach to the promotion of health, including physical activity (see chapter 2), and can be taught within a number of contexts—for example, integrating it into or permeating it through curriculum PE (e.g., during athletics, dance, games, gymnastics, outdoor education and swimming) and teaching it in thematic or topic-based blocks or units of work. Learning outcomes that are integrated into or permeated through curriculum PE should not be lost or allowed to take second place to other learning (e.g., skill development, tactical understanding), and outcomes addressed through topics or projects should relate closely to the content and delivery of curriculum PE and related subjects (e.g., science).

Sample Health-Related Scheme of Work for 7- to 11-Year-Olds

The health-related learning identified in this example spans four academic years and is taught through a combination of curriculum PE and a topic-based project called Be Healthy and Active. This learning sits within a whole-school approach to health that prioritises the promotion of physical activity, healthy eating and emotional well-being.

HEALTH-RELATED LEARNING CATEGORY: SAFETY ISSUES

HEALTH-RELATED LEARNING OUTCOMES

- Explain the need for safety rules and practices (e.g., adopting good posture at all times; being hygienic; changing clothes and having a wash after energetic activity; wearing footwear as appropriate; following rules; protecting against cold weather; avoiding sunburn; lifting safely; using space sensibly [not bumping into others]).

- Identify the purpose of warming up and of cooling down and recognise and describe the parts of a warm-up and of a cool-down: exercises for the joints (e.g., arm circles), whole-body activities (e.g., jogging, skipping without a rope) and stretches for either the whole body (e.g., reaching long and tall) or parts of the body (e.g., lower-leg or calf muscles).

HEALTH-RELATED LEARNING CONTEXT

These learning outcomes are taught in PE lessons and cross-referenced to PSHE education in which pupils are taught about keeping themselves and others safe (e.g., protecting themselves from dehydration and sunburn) (PSHE Association, 2014).

METHODS OF ASSESSING HEALTH-RELATED LEARNING OUTCOMES

- Ask pupils questions such as the following:
  - Why is good posture important?
  - Why do we change for activity?
  - Why do we wash after energetic activity?
  - Why is it sensible to wear trainers for activities such as jumping and playing games?
  - Discuss with a partner some rules in PE or sport. Why do we have rules?
  - Talk with a partner about how to avoid feeling cold in the winter.
  - Talk with a partner about how to avoid getting sunburnt.
  - Why do we warm up?
  - What is a cool-down for?
  - Talk with a partner about the types of exercises included in a warm-up (or cool-down).
- Involve pupils in active assessment tasks such as the following:
  - Show me how to walk with good posture.
  - Demonstrate how to lift something heavy.
  - Show me some activities to warm up your whole body.
  - Show me an exercise for your shoulders (or hips).
  - Demonstrate a whole-body stretch.

HEALTH-RELATED LEARNING CATEGORY: EXERCISE EFFECTS

HEALTH-RELATED LEARNING OUTCOMES

- Explain and feel the short-term effects of exercise.
  - Breathing rate and depth increase to provide more oxygen to working muscles.
  - Heart rate increases to pump more oxygen to working muscles.
  - Temperature increases because working muscles produce energy in the form of heat; as that heat is transferred to the body's surface (skin) to control body temperature, the skin can become moist, sticky and sweaty.
  - Appearance can become flushed due to blood vessels widening and getting closer to the surface of the skin.
  - Feelings and moods can vary (e.g., having fun, feeling good among friends).
- Explain that the body needs a certain amount of energy every day in the form of food and drink in order to function properly (e.g., for normal growth, development and daily living) and that body fat increases if more calories are taken in than are needed

(e.g., for breathing, growing, sleeping, eating, moving, exercising).

HEALTH-RELATED LEARNING CONTEXT

These learning outcomes are taught in PE lessons and cross-referenced to learning in science.

METHODS OF ASSESSING HEALTH-RELATED LEARNING OUTCOMES

- Ask pupils questions such as the following:
  - How does your breathing change when you are active? Why does it do this?
  - Why does your heart rate change when you are active?
  - What happens to your body temperature when you are active, and why?
  - Why do we sometimes sweat when we are active?
  - Talk with a partner about why our appearance can change when we do energetic activity.
  - How do you feel when you are active (e.g., jogging, dancing, playing games)?

- What does the body need energy for? Where does this energy come from?
- How much food and drink does the body need?
- What can happen if the body has too much or too little food and drink?

- Involve pupils in active assessment tasks such as the following:
  - Show me how you can increase your heart rate and breathing rate.
  - Demonstrate some activities that make you warm (or hot).

HEALTH-RELATED LEARNING CATEGORY: HEALTH BENEFITS

HEALTH-RELATED LEARNING OUTCOMES

- Explain that activity strengthens bones and muscles (including the heart) and helps keep joints flexible.
- Explain that activity can help one feel good about oneself and can be fun and social (e.g., involves sharing experiences and cooperating with others).
- Explain that regular activity permits one to perform daily activities more easily.
- Explain that being active helps one maintain a healthy body weight.

HEALTH-RELATED LEARNING CONTEXT

These learning outcomes are addressed within the Be Healthy and Active project that covers related PSHE education (e.g., learning how to make informed choices and beginning to understand the concept of a balanced lifestyle) (PSHE Association, 2014) and are cross-referenced to learning in PE.

METHODS OF ASSESSING HEALTH-RELATED LEARNING OUTCOMES

- Ask pupils questions such as the following:
  - How does being active strengthen bones and muscles?
  - How can being active help you in everyday life?
  - How does activity help you achieve and maintain a healthy weight?
  - Talk with a partner about activities that you like, how they make you feel and why you like them.
  - Name some activities in which you must work together to do well.
- Involve pupils in active assessment tasks such as the following:
  - Show me an activity that strengthens bones and muscles.
  - Demonstrate exercises that help keep your joints flexible.

HEALTH-RELATED LEARNING CATEGORY: ACTIVITY PROMOTION

HEALTH-RELATED LEARNING OUTCOMES

- Monitor their current levels of activity (e.g., daily, twice weekly).
- Identify when, where and how they can be active, both in school and outside of school.
- Make decisions about which physical activities they enjoy and explain that individuals have different feelings about the types and amounts of activity they do.
- Use opportunities to be active for 30 to 60 minutes a day (with rest periods as necessary), including lessons, playtimes and club activities.

HEALTH-RELATED LEARNING CONTEXT

These learning outcomes are addressed within the Be Healthy and Active project and cross-referenced to learning in PE. In particular, they align with a whole-school approach to health, including the promotion of physical activity. Information about activity opportunities on offer in the school and in the local community is communicated to pupils and their families via newsletters, posters, parent mail, parent consultations and assemblies. In addition, the Where to Be Active section of the school website advertises physical activity opportunities at school and within a five-mile radius of the school to connect and support pupils (and families) involved in these activities.

METHODS OF ASSESSING HEALTH-RELATED LEARNING OUTCOMES

- Observe informal activity before and after school and during breaks and lunchtimes.
- Record involvement in formal activities and clubs before, during and after school.
- Have pupils keep an activity diary for one school day and one weekend day, recording all activity they do both at school and outside of school.
- Have pupils pair up and share their activity diaries; they should describe how much activity they did each day, where they did it and with whom. Were they active for an hour a day on these days?

- Discuss how to fit an hour of activity into a day. Ask pupils questions such as the following:
  - When and where can you be active, both in school and outside of school?
- Talk with a partner about which activities you enjoy and which are your favourites. Are there any activities that you do not like so much? If so, what are they, and what do you not like about them?
- Involve pupils in active assessment tasks such as the following:
  - Show me where I can find out about activities outside of school.
  - Mime one of your favourite activities (without equipment)
  - Form a circle and take turns miming your favourite activities; after each mime, everyone copies it.

Medium-term plans for health-related learning generally take the form of units or blocks of work that last for a school term (usually 10 to 14 weekly lessons) or part of a term (usually 4 to 7 weekly lessons). This learning is likely to be within the subject of PE or in thematic or topic-based (or project-based) units or blocks of work with titles such as Be Healthy and Active.

Sample Health-Related Unit of Work for 7- to 11-Year-Olds

The following example presents a six-lesson, topic-based unit called Be Healthy and Active and outlines learning outcomes for selected health benefits and activity promotion for 9- and 10-year-olds. It also covers learning activities to address the outcomes, as well as suggested methods for assessing pupils' learning. The learning in this unit is cross-referenced to related learning in PE.

HEALTH-RELATED LEARNING OUTCOMES: LESSONS 1 AND 2

HEALTH BENEFITS

- Explain that activity strengthens bones and muscles (including the heart) and helps keep joints flexible.
- Explain that activity can help one feel good about oneself and can be fun and social (e.g., sharing experiences and cooperating with others).
- Explain that regular activity permits one to perform daily activities more easily.

HEALTH-RELATED LEARNING ACTIVITIES

- Ask: How does being active affect your heart?

Prompt pupils to think about the heart as a muscle that is made to work during activity, which helps it become more efficient.

- Ask: How does being active affect your bones and muscles?

Prompt pupils to think about activity helping bones and muscles become stronger and, over time, able to work harder and for longer.

- Ask: How does being active affect your joints?

Prompt pupils to think about activity helping joints be more supple, which improves flexibility (i.e., range of movement around joints).

- Ask pupils to show you some activities that make the heart work harder. Encourage them to think of whole-body activities (which use more muscles), such as walking, jogging, skipping, hopping, galloping and moving to music.

    Allow pupils to choose some of these activities and do them with friends or other peers for a set period of time.

- Afterwards, ask: How did you feel about the activities you chose to do? What did you enjoy about them? Why did they make you feel good or happy?

ASSESSMENT OF HEALTH-RELATED LEARNING

- Towards the end of the unit of work, ask pupils questions such as the following:

  – How does being active strengthen bones and muscles?

  – How can being active help you in everyday life?

  – Talk with a partner about activities that you like, how they make you feel, and why you like them.

  – Name some activities in which you must work together to do well.

- Towards the end of the unit of work, involve pupils in active assessment tasks such as the following:

  – Show me an activity that strengthens bones and muscles.

  – Demonstrate exercises that help keep your joints flexible.

HEALTH-RELATED LEARNING OUTCOMES: LESSONS 3 AND 4

ACTIVITY PROMOTION

- Identify when, where and how they can be active, both in and outside of school.
- Make decisions about which physical activities they enjoy and explain that individuals have different feelings about the types and amounts of activity they do.

HEALTH-RELATED LEARNING ACTIVITIES

- Ask: Think of all the ways in which you can be active in school, including travelling to and from school.

    Prompt pupils to consider walking or scooting to and from school, participating in informal activities (in the hall or playground) before school and during breaks and lunchtimes, and participating in formal activities and clubs before and after school and during lunchtimes.

    Encourage pupils to share with a partner what activities they do at school, with whom, and what they think of them. Discuss where to find out about and how to join in with informal activities in school.

- Ask: Think of all the ways you can be active outside of school.

    Prompt pupils to consider walking or scooting to and from home, participating in informal activities (e.g., playing with friends) after school, and taking part in formal activities and clubs after school and at the weekends.

    Encourage pupils to share with a partner what activities they do outside of school, with whom, and what they think of them. Discuss where to find out about and how to join in with activities outside of school.

- Over two lessons, involve pupils in a range of activities, such as skipping and performing exercises to music. Pupils can be taught specific moves (with and without a skipping rope) and then encouraged to put them into a simple routine that can be repeated and performed to music.

- Afterwards, ask: Which activities did you enjoy most? What did you like about them? Why do you think there are different preferences among you?

ASSESSMENT OF HEALTH-RELATED LEARNING

- Towards the end of the unit of work, ask pupils questions such as the following:

– When and where can you be active in school and outside of school?

– Talk with a partner about which activities you enjoy and which are your favourites. Are there any activities that you do not like so much? If so, what are they, and what do you not like about them?

– Tell a partner what activities you do at school, with whom, and what you think of them.

• Towards the end of the unit of work, involve pupils in active assessment tasks such as the following:

– Show me where I can find out about activities outside of school.

– Mime one of your favourite activities (without equipment).

– Form a circle and take turns miming your favourite activities; after each mime, everyone copies it.

HEALTH-RELATED LEARNING OUTCOMES: LESSONS 5 AND 6

ACTIVITY PROMOTION

• Monitor their current levels of activity (e.g., daily, twice weekly).

• Use opportunities to be active for 30 to 60 minutes a day (with rest periods as necessary), including lessons, playtimes and club activities.

HEALTH-RELATED LEARNING ACTIVITIES

• Ask pupils to describe how active they are— for example, very active (all or most days), active (some days), not very active (now and again, or just in PE lessons).

• Ask pupils to keep an activity diary for one school day and one weekend day (for sample activity diaries suitable for this age group, see the web resource for chapter 5). Ask them to record all activity that they do, both at school and outside of school. Talk them through how to complete the activity diary and when to do it.

• Afterwards, ask pupils to show a partner their activity diary and tell them how much activity they did each day, where they did it, and with whom. Ask them to add up the amount of activity time for each of the two days. Were they active for an hour a day on these days?

• Involve pupils in a discussion about how to fit an hour of activity into each day. Remind them about activity opportunities in school and in the local area and about how to find this information.

ASSESSMENT OF HEALTH-RELATED LEARNING

• Where possible during the unit of work, do the following:

– Observe the pupils' informal activity (e.g., in the hall or playground) before and after school and during breaks and lunchtimes.

– Record pupils' involvement in formal activities and clubs before, during and after school.

• Ask pupils to keep an activity diary for one school day and one weekend day, recording all activity that they do, both at school and outside of school.

• In pairs, ask pupils to show a partner their activity diary and discuss how much activity they did each day, where, and with whom. Were they active for an hour a day on these days?

• Involve pupils in a discussion about how to fit an hour of activity into a day.

Short-term plans for health-related learning generally take the form of lesson plans with specific health-related learning outcomes that sit within units or blocks of work. The following example is a lesson plan for 10- and 11-year-olds that outlines selected health-related learning outcomes (focused on cooling down) permeated through an athletics (running) unit of work, as well as learning activities to address the outcomes and suggested methods of assessing the learning.

HEALTH-RELATED LEARNING OUTCOMES

SAFETY ISSUES

- Identify the purpose of a cool-down, and recognise and describe parts of a cool-down—for example, gentle whole-body activities (e.g., jogging, walking) and stretches for the whole body (e.g., reaching long and tall) or parts of the body (e.g., lower-leg or calf muscles).

HEALTH-RELATED LEARNING ACTIVITIES

- Lead the pupils through a warm-up suitable for running, involving mobility exercises for the shoulders and ankles, knee lifts on the spot, walking and jogging, and whole-body stretches (reaching long and tall). During the warm-up, recap prior learning about the purpose of a warm-up and the types of activities included in a warm-up.
- Afterwards, involve the pupils in a series of running activities such as the following:
  - Running 'through the gears' by increasing gradually from first gear (easy jogging) to fifth gear (running very fast).
  - Running as fast as they can for three seconds.
- Next, teach the pupils about good running technique (e.g., head still, face forward, arms driving backward and forward, legs moving as quickly as possible).
- Then engage the pupils in another series of running activities, such as the following:
  - Run as fast as they can for three seconds, trying to run faster and farther than before.
  - Increase the running time to five seconds.
  - Repeat the preceding task several times, focusing on good technique and aiming to run faster and farther than before.
- Afterwards, ask: What do we do after energetic activity to recover? (Sample answer: keep moving slowly and stretch the muscles.)
- Lead the pupils in performing a series of low-intensity exercises, such as walking, knee lifts and side steps. During this sequence, ask: What do we call this? (Recovering from energetic activity, or cooling down.)

- Ask: What types of exercises are included in a cool-down? (Slow activities, such as walking and easy jogging, plus stretches.) Inform pupils that these types of exercises help the joints, bones, muscles (including the heart), lungs and mind recover from energetic activity.
- Ask: How do you feel now? (Better, cooler, not so out of breath, OK or good.)
- Ask pupils to perform some whole-body stretches, such as reaching long and tall and reaching wide with their arms and legs. Teach them a calf stretch and explain that the calf muscles work hard when sprinting and that stretching them lengthens the muscle fibres, thus helping them recover from their hard work.

ASSESSMENT OF HEALTH-RELATED LEARNING

- Ask the following:
  - Why do we cool down?
  - Talk with a partner about the types of exercises included in a cool-down.
  - Show me some activities to slow or cool down your body.
  - Demonstrate a whole-body stretch.

A worksheet associated with this lesson is provided in the web resource for this chapter.

Why Is It Cool to Cool Down?

What do we do after energetic activity to recover?	
Why do we cool down?	
What types of activities help you recover and cool down?	
How do you feel after you have done a cool-down?	

Show me some activities to cool down your body.

Demonstrate two whole-body stretches.

Summary

If you take a structured, progressive approach to children's learning about leading a healthy, active lifestyle, then you can engage them with this important aspect of the curriculum in a way that is comprehensive, coherent and meaningful. This sort of approach needs to be evident at all stages of schooling and be accessible to every pupil. A good way to start is to develop health-related learning plans that include relevant outcomes for successive age groups. The learning can then be organised, taught and assessed in multiple ways and can incorporate the monitoring of children's health, activity and fitness through methods that are developmentally appropriate and pedagogically desirable.

Health-Related Learning for 11- to 14-Year-Olds

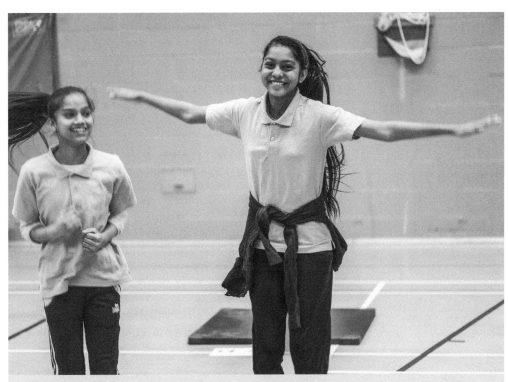

Chapter Objectives

After reading this chapter, you will be able to

- ▶ identify appropriate health-related learning outcomes and contexts for 11- to 14-year-olds;
- ▶ implement a variety of approaches to assess the health-related learning of 11- to 14-year-olds;
- ▶ describe methods of monitoring the health, activity and fitness of 11- to 14-year-olds; and
- ▶ create long-, medium- and short-term plans for health-related learning for 11- to 14-year-olds.

Secondary-school children need to learn about leading a healthy, active lifestyle in a manner that is structured, progressive and accessible to all pupils. The learning can be organised in multiple ways, including activity-based units of work in PE and separate health-related units of work in PE. This chapter proposes health-related learning approaches for 11- to 14-year-olds and provides you with guidance for assessing pupils' learning. It also suggests methods for monitoring the health, activity and fitness of 11- to 14-year-olds, such as health behaviour questionnaires, activity diaries and questionnaires, heart rate monitors, pedometers and accelerometers, and developmentally appropriate fitness tests. Finally, the chapter provides sample schemes, units of work and lesson plans to help you create health-related learning plans that ensure a comprehensive, coherent and meaningful approach to this important aspect of the curriculum.

Health-Related Learning Outcomes and Contexts

As detailed in chapter 3, approaches to health-related learning for the 5- to 16-year-old age group were debated and agreed on in England in 2000 by a working group comprising representatives of national PE, sport and health organisations. Table 10.1 presents specific health-related learning outcomes for 11- to 14-year-olds; the outcomes are presented in four categories—safety issues, exercise effects, health benefits and activity promotion—to help clarify the scope and progression of the learning.

The learning content detailed in table 10.1 can be taught in a number of contexts. One approach is to integrate it into or permeate it through activity-based units of work in PE (e.g., athletics, dance, games, gymnastics, outdoor education and swimming lessons). Another approach is to teach it in separate thematic units of work in PE with a title such as Health-Related Exercise or Action for Health. A third option is to combine the first two approaches. Limitations in these approaches (discussed in chapter 3) can be addressed by ensuring that learning outcomes integrated into or permeated through activity-based units of work in PE are not lost and do not take second place to other learning (e.g., skill development, tactical understanding, choreography). In addition, learning outcomes taught in separate health-related units of work in PE should be connected closely with the rest of the PE curriculum and with the content and delivery of related subjects (e.g., science; food technology; personal, social, health and economic [PSHE] education) and extracurricular and community activity experiences.

More specifically, the learning outcomes related to safety issues can be permeated through activity-based units of work in PE. The learning outcomes related to exercise effects and to health benefits can be either permeated through activity-based units of work in PE or taught in additional health-related units of work. Explicit links should be made with PSHE education for this age group, which includes learning about the benefits of physical activity and exercise and the importance of balancing work, leisure and exercise (PSHE Association, 2014). The learning outcomes related to activity promotion can be either permeated through PE units of work or taught in additional health-related units of work. Here again, explicit links should be made with PSHE education for this age group, which in this case includes helping pupils learn to recognise and manage influences on their choices about exercise (PSHE Association, 2014).

To ensure alignment with a whole-school approach to health, including the promotion of physical activity, information about activity opportunities on offer in the school and in the local community can be communicated to pupils and their families in a multitude of ways (e.g., newsletters, posters, parent mail, parent consultations, assemblies). In addition, the school website can have a dedicated Where to Be Active section highlighting physical activity opportunities both at school and within a five-mile radius of the school; this section can also be used to connect and support pupils (and families) involved in these activities.

Assessing Health-Related Learning

Health-related learning can be assessed via written, verbal and active responses to questions, tasks and tests. In terms of focus, assessment can address affective, behavioural and cognitive (ABC) learning outcomes; for more on ABC outcomes, see chapter 3. Affective and behavioural outcomes for 11- to 14-year-olds can be assessed via teacher observation of effort and commitment

TABLE 10.1　Health-Related Learning Outcomes for Ages 11 to 14

Pupils who are 11 to 14 years old can do the following:

Safety issues	• Demonstrate their understanding of safe exercise practices (e.g., tying long hair back and removing jewellery to avoid injury; adopting good posture when sitting, standing and moving; performing exercises with good technique; having a wash or shower following energetic activity; using equipment and facilities with permission and, where necessary, under supervision; administering basic first aid; wearing adequate protection such as goalkeeping gloves and leg pads as appropriate; coping with specific weather conditions, such as using sunscreen to avoid sunburn and drinking fluids to prevent dehydration; following proper procedures for specific activities). • Demonstrate their concern for and understanding of back care by lifting, carrying, placing and using equipment responsibly and with good technique. • Explain why certain exercises and practices are not recommended (e.g., standing toe touches, straight-leg sit-ups, bounces during stretching, flinging movements) and be able to perform safe alternatives (e.g., seated sit-and-reach stretch, curl-up with bent legs, stretches held still, movements performed with control). • Explain the value of preparing for and recovering from activity and the possible consequences of not doing so. • More specifically, explain the purpose of, and plan and perform, each component of a warm-up and of a cool-down (i.e., mobility exercises, whole-body activities, static stretches) both for activity in general (e.g., games, athletics) and for specific activities (e.g., volleyball, high jump, circuit training). • Use good technique in performing developmentally appropriate cardiorespiratory activities, as well as strength and flexibility exercises, for each major muscle group.
Exercise effects	• Explain and monitor a range of short-term effects of exercise on 　• the cardiorespiratory system (e.g., changes in breathing, heart rate, temperature, appearance, feelings, recovery rate and ability to pace oneself and remain within a target zone) and 　• the musculoskeletal system (e.g., increases in muscular strength, endurance and flexibility; improved muscle tone and posture; enhanced functional capacity and sport or dance performance). • Explain that appropriate training can improve fitness and performance and that specific types of activity affect specific aspects of fitness (e.g., running affects cardiorespiratory fitness). • Explain the differences between whole-body activities (e.g., walking, jogging, cycling, dancing, swimming) that help reduce body fat and conditioning exercises (e.g., straight and twisting curl-ups) that improve muscle tone.
Health benefits	• Explain a range of long-term benefits of activity on physical health, such as 　• reduced risk of chronic disease (e.g., heart disease), 　• reduced risk of bone disease (e.g., osteoporosis), 　• reduced risk of some other health conditions (e.g., obesity, back pain) and 　• improved management of some health conditions (e.g., asthma, diabetes, arthritis). • Explain that activity can enhance mental health and social and psychological well-being (e.g., enjoyment of being with friends, increased confidence and self-esteem, decreased anxiety and stress) and that an appropriate balance between work, leisure and exercise promotes good health. • Explain that increasing activity levels and eating a balanced diet can help one maintain a healthy body weight (i.e., energy balance), that the body needs a certain minimum daily energy intake in order to function properly and that strict dieting and excessive exercising can damage one's health. • Explain that each activity area (athletics, dance, games, gymnastics, swimming and outdoor and adventurous activities) can contribute to physical health and to social and psychological well-being (e.g., can improve stamina, assist weight management, strengthen bones, be enjoyable).
Activity promotion	• Access information about a range of activity opportunities at school, at home and in the local community and identify ways to incorporate activity into their lifestyles (e.g., walking or cycling to school or to meet friends; helping around the home or garden). • Reflect on their activity strengths and preferences and know how to get involved in activities. • Participate in activity of at least moderate intensity for one hour every day (accumulated over the course of a day), including activity that strengthens muscles and bones. • Monitor and evaluate personal activity levels over a period of time (e.g., by keeping an activity diary for four to six weeks and reflecting on the experience).

in PE lessons, as well as participation records for PE lessons and extracurricular activities (using ratings such as excellent, good, satisfactory or adequate, and low or inadequate). Cognitive outcomes can be assessed through question-and-answer episodes and through practical and active tasks. Active assessment tasks are particularly encouraged because they increase activity levels in PE lessons (for more information about active assessment, see chapter 3). Table 10.2 presents a range of methods for assessing the recommended health-related learning outcomes for 11- to 14-year-olds.

TABLE 10.2 Methods of Assessing Health-Related Learning in 11- to 14-Year-Olds

Health-related learning category	Health-related learning outcomes	Methods of assessing health-related learning outcomes

Safety issues	• Demonstrate their understanding of safe exercise practices (e.g., tying long hair back and removing jewellery to avoid injury; adopting good posture when sitting, standing or moving; performing exercises with good technique; having a wash or shower following energetic activity; using equipment and facilities with permission and, where necessary, under supervision; administering basic first aid; wearing adequate protection, such as goalkeeping gloves and leg pads, as appropriate; coping with specific weather conditions, such as using sunscreen to avoid sunburn and drinking fluids to prevent dehydration; following procedures for specific activities).
	• Demonstrate their concern for and understanding of back care by lifting, carrying, placing and using equipment responsibly and with good technique.
	• Explain why certain exercises and practices are not recommended (e.g., standing toe touches, straight-leg sit-ups, bounces during stretches, flinging movements) and be able to perform safe alternatives (e.g., seated sit-and-reach stretch, curl-up with bent legs, stretches held still, movements performed with control).
	• Explain the value of preparing for and recovering from activity and the possible consequences of not doing so.
	• More specifically, explain the purpose of, and plan and perform, each component of a warm-up and of a cool-down (i.e., mobility exercises, whole-body activities, static stretches) for activity in general (e.g., games, athletics) and for specific activities (e.g., volleyball, high jump, circuit training).
	• Use good technique in performing developmentally appropriate cardiorespiratory activities and strength and flexibility exercises for each major muscle group.
		• Ask pupils questions such as these:
		  • Why should long hair be tied back in PE lessons?
		  • Why do we ask you to remove jewellery in PE lessons?
		  • Why should you wash or shower following energetic activity?
		  • Discuss with a partner what 'good posture' means and guide your partner to walk with good posture.
		  • Talk with a partner about what you would do if someone fell and was in pain.
		  • Why is it important to drink water when exercising in hot weather?
		  • How should you protect yourself from the sun?
		  • State three rules that help keep athletics throwing events safe.
		  • Talk with a partner about how to safely lift something heavy.
		  • How does warming up help your body prepare for energetic activity?
		  • What types of exercises should be included in a warm-up, and why?
		  • Why is it important to cool down after very vigorous activity?
		  • What types of exercises should be included in a cool-down, and why?
		  • Talk with a partner about how you should feel after a cool-down.
		• Involve pupils in active assessment tasks such as these:
		  • Show me how to sit, stand and move with good posture.
		  • Demonstrate with a partner how to safely lift a bench or box.
		  • Perform an effective stretch for the hamstrings.
		  • In a small group, design a general warm-up to show to others; include mobility exercises, whole-body activities and static stretches (in that order).
		  • In a small group, design a warm-up to lead others through for the long jump; include mobility exercise, whole-body activities and static stretches relevant to the long jump.

Health-related learning category	Health-related learning outcomes	Methods of assessing health-related learning outcomes

Exercise effects	• Explain and monitor a range of short-term effects of exercise on
	  • the cardiorespiratory system (e.g., changes in breathing, heart rate, temperature, appearance, feelings, recovery rate and ability to pace oneself and remain within a target zone) and
	  • the musculoskeletal system (e.g., increases in muscular strength, endurance and flexibility; improved muscle tone and posture; enhanced functional capacity and sport or dance performance).
	• Explain that appropriate training can improve fitness and performance and that specific types of activity affect specific aspects of fitness (e.g., running affects cardiorespiratory fitness).
	• Explain the differences between whole-body activities (e.g., walking, jogging, cycling, dancing, swimming) that help reduce body fat and conditioning exercises (e.g., straight and twisting curl-ups) that improve muscle tone.
		• Ask pupils questions such as these:
		  • Why does your heart rate increase when you exercise?
		  • What happens to your breathing rate during energetic activity, and why?
		  • How does the body regulate its temperature during exercise?
		  • In what ways can your appearance change when you exercise, and why do these changes occur?
		  • Talk with a partner about exercises you can do to improve your posture.
		  • Match activities to components of fitness (e.g., running develops cardiorespiratory fitness).
		  • Think of and perform six whole-body activities. How do such activities help reduce body fat?
		• Involve pupils in active assessment tasks such as these:
		  • Show me two exercises to develop tone in your abdominal muscles.
		  • Demonstrate how to develop strength and endurance in your chest muscles.
		  • With a partner, perform four whole-body activities to music; put them into a sequence to teach to others.

Health benefits	• Explain a range of long-term benefits of activity on physical health, such as
	  • reduced risk of chronic disease (e.g., heart disease),
	  • reduced risk of bone disease (e.g., osteoporosis),
	  • reduced risk of some other health conditions (e.g., obesity, back pain) and
	  • improved management of some health conditions (e.g., asthma, diabetes, arthritis).
	• Explain that activity can enhance mental health and social and psychological well-being (e.g., enjoyment of being with friends, increased confidence and self-esteem, decreased anxiety and stress) and that an appropriate balance between work, leisure and exercise promotes good health.
	• Explain that increasing activity levels and eating a balanced diet can help one maintain a healthy body weight (i.e., energy balance), that the body needs a certain minimum daily energy intake in order to function properly and that strict dieting and excessive exercising can damage one's health.
	• Explain how each activity area (athletics, dance, games, gymnastics, swimming and outdoor and adventurous activities) can contribute to physical health and to social and psychological well-being (e.g., can improve stamina, assist in weight management, strengthen bones, be enjoyable).
		• Ask pupils questions such as these:
		  • How does being active help reduce your risk of heart disease?
		  • How can activity help prevent you from getting bone conditions such as osteoporosis?
		  • How does activity help individuals with asthma?
		  • In what ways can activity help you feel good?
		  • Name some activities that can calm or relax the body and mind.
		  • Why is it important to maintain balance between work, leisure and exercise?
		  • Explain to a partner what energy balance is.
		  • Why is it essential to have a minimum daily energy intake?
		  • How can strict dieting and excessive exercise affect your body and mind?
		  • In a small group, match activity areas to health benefits (e.g. dance can improve stamina and flexibility, strengthen bones, assist with healthy weight management and be enjoyable).
		• Involve pupils in active assessment tasks such as these:
		  • Mime movements from an activity area and talk about health benefits of this type of activity.
		  • Jog with a partner and chat about how activity can assist with healthy weight management.

(continued)

Table 10.2 *(continued)*

Health-related learning category	Health-related learning outcomes	Methods of assessing health-related learning outcomes

Activity promotion	• Access information about a range of activity opportunities at school, at home and in the local community and identify ways to incorporate activity into their lifestyles (e.g., walking or cycling to school or to meet friends; helping around the home or garden).
	
	• Reflect on their activity strengths and preferences and know how to get involved in activities.
	
	• Participate in activity of at least moderate intensity for a minimum of half an hour and preferably for one hour every day (i.e., 30 to 60 minutes accumulated over the course of a day).
	
	• Participate in activity of at least moderate intensity for one hour every day (accumulated over the course of a day), including activity that strengthens muscles and bones.
	
	• Monitor and evaluate personal activity levels over a period of time (e.g., by keeping an activity diary for four to six weeks and reflecting on the experience).
		• Ask questions such as these:
		  • Tell me five ways to incorporate routine physical activity into your lifestyle.
		  • Discuss with a partner your favourite activities and why you like them.
		  • How much activity should young people do?
		  • What does 'at least moderate intensity' mean?
		  • Give me examples of activities of 'at least moderate intensity'.
		  • Explain to a partner what 'accumulated over the course of a day' means.
		  • Keep an activity diary for four to six weeks; record all the activity that you do and its intensity and duration.
		  • Talk your partner through your activity diary and discuss what it shows about your activity patterns or habits.
		
		• Involve pupils in active assessment tasks such as these:
		  • Show me where you can find information about activity opportunities in the local community.
		  • Demonstrate 'moderate intensity' and then 'vigorous intensity'.
		  • Walk and jog with a partner while talking about activity opportunities at school, at home and in the local community that you are (or have been) involved in.

Monitoring Health, Activity and Fitness

The rationale for monitoring children's health, activity and fitness has been strengthened in recent years both by increased concern about children's physical, mental and social health and by the trend towards sedentary living that marks a more technologically advanced world. These issues are addressed in part I of this book, whereas part II covers developmentally and pedagogically appropriate approaches to monitoring within the curriculum in order to promote healthy, active lifestyles among children. The following examples are appropriate for use with 11- to 14-year-olds.

Monitoring Health

We can help children become more aware of their lifestyles by using health behaviour question-naires that offer a selection of responses (e.g., always, mostly, sometimes, never) to questions such as the following:

• Do you eat a balanced diet that is low(ish) in sugar and fat?

• Do you eat a combined total of five portions of vegetables and fruits each day?

• Do you have a sensible balance between rest, work and play?

• Are you active for about an hour every day?

Chapter 4 provides an example of a health behaviour questionnaire suitable for secondary-age pupils; it can be used to calculate a health score linked to generic feedback such as the following: 'You lead a healthy lifestyle some of the time and will benefit from doing so. However, you should consider leading a healthier lifestyle by improving on a number of your habits'. Engaging children in the process of self-reflection enhances learning and helps children to set measurable targets for improvement. Here are a few sample questions to ask of 11- to 14-year-olds: 'What have you done well on? What can you improve on? What are you able to change about your health? State three actions that you can carry out over the next three months to improve your health.' Additional examples of self-reflection questions are provided in chapter 4.

Responses to these questions can be used to trigger discussions among pupils about ways to lead a healthy lifestyle, as well as relevant barriers and facilitators. When conducting such discussions, be sensitive to the fact that children of all ages (including secondary-age children) have no control over major factors that influence their health—for example, genetics, environment (e.g., pollution, poverty) and family modelling. In addition, they have only partial control over other key factors, including what they eat and drink and how active they are. So, whilst children can learn about leading a healthy lifestyle (and the consequences of not doing so), they should also be aware of which factors influencing their health lie beyond their control and which ones they have some control over. Furthermore, leading a healthy lifestyle can cost more in terms of purchasing healthy foods and drinks and accessing physical activity opportunities (e.g., after-school or holiday clubs) that require payment. As a consequence, children from low-income families may be disadvantaged in comparison with their peers and, where possible, should be offered free or low-cost opportunities to consume healthy meals and drinks and to be active.

Monitoring Activity

As described in chapter 5, children's physical activity can be monitored through a number of methods. One appropriate method for 11- to 14-year-olds involves self-reporting—for example, keeping a physical activity diary for four to six weeks (for examples of activity diaries suitable for this age group, see the web resource for chapter 5). More formal self-report instruments suitable for use with secondary-age children include the Previous Day Physical Activity Recall (PDPAR), the Three-Day Physical Activity Recall (3DPAR), the Physical Activity Questionnaire for Children (PAQ-C) or for Adolescents (PAQ-A), the Youth Risk Behaviour Surveillance System (YRBSS) and the Teen Health Survey. For more information about these instruments, see Trost (2007) and Biddle, Gorely, Pearson, and Bull (2011). Addi-

tional methods suitable for 11- to 14-year-olds include the use of pedometers, accelerometers and heart rate monitors (i.e., chest-strap transmitters paired with a wrist receiver or mobile phone); for a discussion of the advantages and disadvantages of these methods, see chapter 5. In recent years, accelerometers have also been developed into popular wearable electronic devices (e.g., Fitbit) that monitor physical activity and provide additional information and feedback on specific aspects of activity.

You can encourage pupils to reflect on their activity levels by asking questions such as the following: Do you usually take part in 60 minutes or more of moderate to vigorous activity each day? Do you think you should be more active? If yes, what is your physical activity goal? Who or what could help you achieve this goal? (For more examples appropriate for secondary-age children, see the web resource for chapter 5).

You may also want to incorporate questions about sedentary behaviour into discussions about healthy lifestyles. This approach links with the UK-wide physical activity guideline that children and young people should minimise the amount of time spent being sedentary (for more information about this and other guidelines, see chapter 1). Young people's responses to questions such as 'Are you ever sedentary for extended periods of time?' and 'What could you do to reduce the amount of time for which you are sedentary?' can be used to promote discussion about inactivity, its consequences, and ways in which the school environment could encourage less sedentary behaviour.

Whilst obtaining a precise measure of physical activity is important for research purposes, it is less crucial for teachers, whose main concerns relate to the educational value of the monitoring experience and its ease of use, feasibility and cost. From a pedagogical perspective, it is considered more important to ensure that pupils enjoy, learn and benefit from the monitoring experience than to worry unduly about the precision of the method (Cale & Harris, 2009b). This learning can include knowing how to routinely incorporate physical activity into their lifestyles, knowing how to get involved in organised activities and reflecting on their activity strengths and preferences.

Pupils should be encouraged to think of ways in which they could be more physically active at school, at home and in the local community. Their responses can be used to prompt discussion about healthy, active lifestyles, including consideration

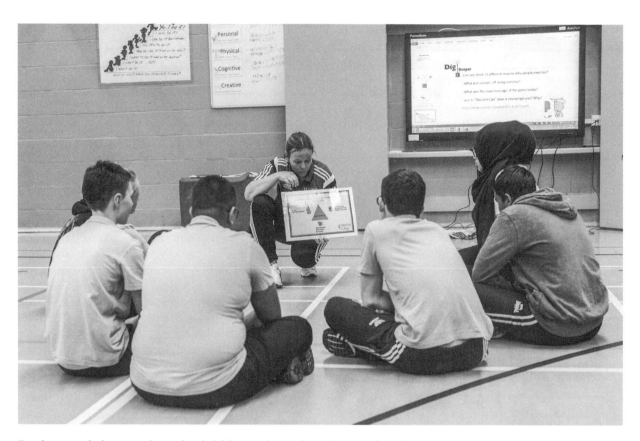

Teachers can help secondary school children to learn about the benefits of being active and how to go about leading healthy, active lifestyles.

of what helps and what hinders their participation in physical activity. Pupils can also be encouraged to discuss and critique visual images in the media in order to challenge common misunderstandings and misconceptions about physical activity—for example, believing that light-intensity activity offers no health benefits and that activity must hurt in order to do any good (see chapter 1 for a discussion of young people's inaccurate and inadequate understandings of health, fitness and physical activity).

Monitoring Fitness

As discussed in chapter 6, fitness testing is controversial in a school setting, and before using it with children we must consider a number of issues and limitations. Fitness monitoring can be considered a valuable component of the curriculum if it is developmentally appropriate; offers a positive, educational experience for all learners; and helps promote healthy, active lifestyles (Association for Physical Education, 2015a, 2015b;

Cale, 2016; Cale & Harris, 2009a, 2009b; Cale, Harris, & Chen, 2014; Lloyd, Colley, & Tremblay, 2010; Rowland, 2007; Silverman, Keating, & Phillips, 2008).

It is not essential for children aged 11 to 14 to be involved in formal fitness testing in order for them to learn that certain activities develop fitness (e.g., dancing improves cardiorespiratory fitness; curl-ups and push-ups improve strength and endurance in specific muscle groups). These associations can be taught in PE lessons, where children learn, for example, that swimming and aerobics help improve their cardiorespiratory fitness, flexibility and muscular strength and endurance.

If you choose to involve 11- to 14-year-olds in formal fitness testing, select the tests carefully and teach them in a positive, supportive setting. Emphasise helping pupils enjoy and learn from the experience and strive to improve on their own personal-best scores. Submaximal tests are recommended for this age group—for example, the step test and the mini bleep test for cardio-

COMMUNITY OF PRACTICE

A number of secondary-school PE teachers in the Midlands who met once a term as a regional group decided to focus on key objectives linked to national curriculum requirements, one of which was 'leading healthy, active lifestyles'. In their meetings during one particular year, they discussed issues associated with promoting active lifestyles and shared various ideas and resources. Some of the teachers had been involved in a PAL (promoting active lifestyles) project during their teacher training course and therefore were able to critique traditional approaches in this area (e.g., those dominated by fitness testing and sport training) and present alternative approaches.

Specifically, these teachers distributed professional and academic journal articles on the chosen topic and shared resources, such as an infographic addressing the recommendation to engage in one hour per day of physical activity for health, a model of the active school, and selected Change4Life and This Girl Can materials for use with pupils and parents. They also showed colleagues resources that they had learned about as part of the PAL project, such as calorie cards (each picturing a food, indicating its calorie count, and suggesting activities to use that number of calories) and circuit cards (focused on learning about posture, aerobic activity, impact and intensity).

Discussion points: Would you find it useful to discuss issues and share resources with teachers from schools in your region? What could you share with them related to promoting active lifestyles?

This supportive community of practice helped the teachers adopt a more critical, explicit and effective approach to promoting active lifestyles in PE in their schools. They reported that sharing ideas and resources in the regional meetings proved to be an invaluable form of professional development that led to positive changes in both curricular and extracurricular programmes, thus benefiting their teaching colleagues and pupils.

Discussion points: What advantages do you see in this approach to professional development? Are there any possible disadvantages to this approach? If so, how might they be minimised?

respiratory fitness and differentiated versions of exercises for muscular strength and endurance (e.g., curl-up, push-up). The web resource for chapter 6 provides descriptions of these tests, as well as recommendations to consider before, during and after implementing them. Once fitness testing is completed, ask pupils to reflect on the experience and on their scores. The web resource for chapter 6 provides examples of appropriate questions for secondary-age children, such as the following: What component of fitness did each test measure, and why is each component important? Talk about your results: Can you explain them? What might have affected them? How would you feel about doing the tests again in two or three months?

All children aged 11 to 14 years should be helped to understand that fitness is developed by being physically active and is associated with good health. This message is consistent with the goal of influencing the process (being active) rather than the product (fitness) (Cale & Harris,

2009b). In addition, pupils can be encouraged to discuss and critique images from the media relating to fitness in order to challenge any misunderstandings and misconceptions that they may have about fitness—for example, believing that fitness is predominantly about one's weight and physical appearance (see chapter 1 for a discussion of young people's inaccurate and inadequate understandings of health, fitness and physical activity).

Health-Related Learning Plans for 11- to 14-Year Olds

Long-term health-related plans generally take the form of a scheme of work over a number of years. In the case of 11- to 14-year-olds, the duration of the scheme of work is three academic years. Ideally, the health-related learning should sit within a whole-school approach to the promotion of health (see chapter 2) and can be taught within a number of contexts—for example, integrating it into activity-based units of work and separate thematic health-related units of work in PE. Learning outcomes that are integrated into or permeated through activity-based units of work in PE should not be lost or allowed to take second place to other learning (e.g., skill development, tactical understanding, choreography), and outcomes addressed though separate health-related units of work in PE should relate closely to the rest of the PE curriculum and to the content and delivery of related subjects (e.g., science, food technology, PSHE education).

Sample Health-Related Scheme of Work for 11- to 14-Year-Olds

The health-related learning identified in this example spans three academic years and is taught through activity-based units of work in PE in combination with separate, thematic health-related units of work in PE called Action for Health. This learning sits within a whole-school approach to health that aims to achieve healthy lifestyles for the entire school population by developing a supportive environment that is conducive to promoting health through the curriculum, the environment and the community.

HEALTH-RELATED LEARNING CATEGORY: SAFETY ISSUES

HEALTH-RELATED LEARNING OUTCOMES

- Demonstrate their understanding of safe exercise practices (e.g., tying long hair back and removing jewellery to avoid injury; adopting good posture when sitting, standing or moving; performing exercises with good technique; having a wash or shower following energetic activity; using equipment and facilities with permission and, where necessary, under supervision; administering basic first aid; wearing adequate protection, such as goalkeeping gloves and leg pads, as appropriate; coping with specific weather conditions, such as using sunscreen to avoid sunburn and drinking fluids to prevent dehydration; following proper procedures for specific activities).

- Demonstrate their concern for and understanding of back care by lifting, carrying, placing and using equipment responsibly and with good technique

- Explain why certain exercises and practices are not recommended (e.g., standing toe touches, straight-leg sit-ups, bounces during stretches, flinging movements) and be able to perform safe alternatives (e.g., seated sit-and-reach stretch, curl-up with bent legs, stretches held still, movements performed with control).

- Explain the value of purposefully preparing for and recovering from activity and the possible consequences of not doing so.

- More specifically, explain the purpose of, and plan and perform, each component of a warm-up and of a cool-down (i.e., mobility exercises, whole-body activities, static stretches) for activity in general (e.g., games, athletics) and for specific activities (e.g., volleyball, high jump, circuit training).

- Use good technique in performing developmentally appropriate cardiorespiratory activities, as well as strength and flexibility exercises, for each major muscle group.

HEALTH-RELATED LEARNING CONTEXT

These learning outcomes are taught in activity-based units of work in curriculum PE with explicit links to safety issues that arise in extracurricular and community settings (e.g., demonstrating safe exercise practices, preparing for and recovering from activity, performing activities and exercises with good technique).

METHODS OF ASSESSING HEALTH-RELATED LEARNING OUTCOMES

Ask pupils questions such as the following:
- Why should long hair be tied back in PE lessons?
- Why do we ask you to remove jewellery in PE lessons?
- Why should you wash or shower following energetic activity?

- Discuss with a partner what 'good posture' means and guide your partner to walk with good posture.
- Talk with a partner about what you would do if someone fell and was in pain.
- Why is it important to drink water when exercising in hot weather?
- How should you protect yourself from the sun?
- State three rules that help keep athletics throwing events safe.
- Talk with a partner about how to safely lift something heavy.
- How does warming up help your body prepare for energetic activity?
- What types of exercises should be included in a warm-up, and why?
- Why is it important to cool down after very vigorous activity?

- What types of exercises should be included in a cool-down, and why?
- Talk with a partner about how you should feel after a cool-down.

Involve pupils in active assessment tasks such as the following:

- Show me how to sit, stand and move with good posture.
- Demonstrate with a partner how to safely lift a bench or box.
- Perform an effective stretch for the hamstrings.
- In a small group, design a general warm-up to show to others; include mobility exercises, whole-body activities and static stretches (in that order).
- In a small group, design a warm-up for the long jump to lead others through; include mobility exercise, whole-body activities and static stretches relevant to the long jump.

HEALTH-RELATED LEARNING CATEGORY: EXERCISE EFFECTS

HEALTH-RELATED LEARNING OUTCOMES

- Explain and monitor a range of short-term effects of exercise on
  - the cardiovascular system (e.g., changes in breathing and heart rate, temperature, appearance, feelings, recovery rate and ability to pace oneself and remain within a target zone) and
  - the musculoskeletal system (e.g., increases in muscular strength and endurance and flexibility; improved muscle tone and posture; enhanced functional capacity and sport or dance performance).
- Explain that appropriate training can improve fitness and performance and that specific types of activity affect specific aspects of fitness (e.g., running affects cardiorespiratory fitness).
- Explain the differences between whole-body activities (e.g., walking, jogging, cycling, dancing, swimming) that help reduce body fat and conditioning exercises (e.g., straight and twisting curl-ups) that improve muscle tone.

HEALTH-RELATED LEARNING CONTEXT

These learning outcomes are taught in activity-based and health-related units of work in curriculum PE with explicit links to related learning in PSHE, science and food technology.

METHODS OF ASSESSING HEALTH-RELATED LEARNING OUTCOMES

Ask pupils questions such as the following:

- Why does your heart rate increase when you exercise?
- What happens to your breathing rate during energetic activity, and why?
- How does the body regulate its temperature during exercise?
- In what ways can your appearance change when you exercise, and why?
- Talk with a partner about exercises you can do to improve your posture.
- Match activities to components of fitness (e.g., running develops cardiorespiratory fitness).
- Perform six whole-body activities; how do these types of activities help reduce body fat?

Involve pupils in active assessment tasks such as the following:

- Show me two exercises to develop tone in your abdominal muscles.

- Demonstrate how to develop the strength and endurance of your chest muscles.
- With a partner, perform four whole-body activities to music; put them into a sequence to teach to others.

HEALTH-RELATED LEARNING CATEGORY: HEALTH BENEFITS

HEALTH-RELATED LEARNING OUTCOMES

- Explain a range of long-term benefits of activity for physical health, such as
  - reduced risk of chronic disease (e.g., heart disease),
  - reduced risk of bone disease (e.g., osteoporosis),
  - reduced risk of some other health conditions (e.g., obesity, back pain) and
  - improved management of some health conditions (e.g., asthma, diabetes, arthritis).
- Explain that activity can enhance mental health and social and psychological well-being (e.g., enjoyment of being with friends; increased confidence and self-esteem; decreased anxiety and stress) and that an appropriate balance between work, leisure and exercise promotes good health.
- Explain that increasing activity levels and eating a balanced diet can help one maintain a healthy body weight (i.e., energy balance), that the body needs a certain minimum daily energy intake in order to function properly and that strict dieting and excessive exercising can damage one's health.
- Explain how each activity area (athletics, dance, games, gymnastics, swimming and outdoor and adventurous activities) can contribute to physical health and to social and psychological well-being (e.g., can improve stamina, assist in weight management, strengthen bones, be enjoyable).

HEALTH-RELATED LEARNING CONTEXT

These learning outcomes are taught in health-related units of work in PE called Action for Health with explicit links to learning in activity-based units of work in PE and in PSHE.

METHODS OF ASSESSING HEALTH-RELATED LEARNING OUTCOMES

Ask pupils questions such as the following:

- How does being active help reduce your risk of heart disease?
- How can activity help prevent you from getting bone conditions such as osteoporosis?
- How does activity help individuals with asthma?
- How can activity help individuals feel good?
- Name some activities that can calm or relax the body and mind.
- Why is it important to balance work, leisure and exercise?
- Explain to a partner what energy balance is.
- Why is it essential to have a minimum daily energy intake?
- How can strict dieting and excessive exercise affect your body and mind?
- In a small group, match activity areas to health benefits (e.g., dance can improve stamina and flexibility, strengthen bones, assist with healthy weight management and be enjoyable).

Involve pupils in active assessment tasks such as the following:

- Mime movements from an activity area and talk about health benefits of this area.
- Jog with a partner and chat about how activity can assist with healthy weight management.

HEALTH-RELATED LEARNING CATEGORY: ACTIVITY PROMOTION

HEALTH-RELATED LEARNING OUTCOMES

- Access information about a range of activity opportunities at school, at home and in the local community and identify ways to incorporate activity into their lifestyles (e.g., walking or cycling to school or to meet friends; helping around the home or garden).
- Reflect on their activity strengths and preferences and know how to get involved in activities.
- Participate in activity of at least moderate intensity for one hour every day (accumulated over the course of a day), including activity that strengthens muscles and bones.
- Monitor and evaluate personal activity levels over a period of time (e.g., by keeping an activity diary for four to six weeks and reflecting on the experience).

HEALTH-RELATED LEARNING CONTEXT

These learning outcomes are addressed in health-related units of work in PE called Action for Health with explicit links to learning in activity-based units of work in PE and in PSHE.

METHODS OF ASSESSING HEALTH-RELATED LEARNING OUTCOMES

Ask questions such as the following:

- Tell me five ways to incorporate routine physical activity into your lifestyle.
- Discuss with a partner your favourite activities and why you like them.
- How much activity should young people do?
- What does 'at least moderate intensity' mean?
- Give me examples of activities that are of 'at least moderate intensity'.
- Explain to a partner what 'accumulated over the course of a day' means.
- Keep an activity diary for four to six weeks; record all of the activity you do, as well as its intensity and duration.
- Talk your partner through your activity diary and discuss what it shows about your activity patterns or habits.

Involve pupils in active assessment tasks such as the following:

- Show me where you can find information about activity opportunities in the local community.
- Demonstrate 'moderate intensity' and then 'vigorous intensity'.
- Walk and jog with a partner while talking about activity opportunities at school, at home and in the local community that you are (or have been) involved in.

Medium-term plans for health-related learning generally take the form of units of work over the course of a school term (usually 10 to 14 weekly lessons) or parts of a term (usually 4 to 7 weekly lessons). These units of work are likely to be within the subject of PE (activity based and health related) with explicit links to learning in related subjects such as PSHE education, science and food technology.

Sample Health-Related Unit of Work for 11- to 14-Year-Olds

The following example presents a six-lesson, topic-based unit called Action for Heart Health and outlines learning outcomes for selected exercise effects and health benefits for 11- and 12-year-olds. It also covers learning activities to address the outcomes, as well as suggested methods for assessing pupils' learning. The learning in this unit is cross-referenced to related learning in activity-based units of work in PE.

HEALTH-RELATED LEARNING OUTCOMES: LESSONS 1 AND 2

EXERCISE EFFECTS

- Explain and monitor a range of short-term effects of exercise on
  - the cardiovascular system (e.g., changes in breathing, heart rate, temperature, appearance, feelings, recovery rate and ability to pace oneself and remain within a target zone) and
  - musculoskeletal system (e.g., increases in muscular strength, endurance and flexibility; improved muscle tone and posture; enhanced functional capacity and sport or dance performance).
- Explain that appropriate training can improve fitness and performance and that specific types of activity affect specific aspects of fitness (e.g., running affects cardiorespiratory fitness).

HEALTH-RELATED LEARNING ACTIVITIES

- Involve pupils in a card game in which they pick up a playing card from the centre of the area and go to different corners or quarters to perform specific exercises for each suit—for example, knee lifts (with or without jumps) for clubs, step-backs or scissor jumps for diamonds, fast walking or jogging for hearts, and sidesteps or astride jumps for spades. The number of exercises performed is determined by the number on the card. After each go, pupils return to the centre, pick up another card and repeat the process; this pattern continues for up to five minutes. The activity can be performed to lively background music.

- After the card game, ask pupils to talk in pairs or small groups about the changes they noticed while exercising. Prompt them to think about changes to heart rate, breathing rate, temperature, appearance and feelings. Facilitate sharing of their responses with the class.

- Next, ask pupils to discuss in pairs or small groups the reasons for the changes they experienced (e.g., heart and breathing rate increase to get oxygenated blood to the working muscles; appearance changes as blood vessels dilate and come closer to the skin's surface, thus giving a flushed look).

Facilitate sharing of pupils' reasons with the class.

- Involve pupils in a posture circuit—that is, a planned sequence of exercises to improve posture. For example, station 1 might involve curl-ups (to address the rectus abdominis), station 2 might involve back raises (erector spinae), station 3 might involve leg raises (gluteus maximus), station 4 might involve twisting curl-ups (obliques) and station 5 might involve shoulder squeezes (trapezius). Each station is equipped with resource cards that show visual images of up to three differentiated versions of the relevant exercise. The exercises can be performed for one minute at each station, and the circuit can be performed to background music.

- During the posture circuit, prompt pupils to think about which muscles are working in each exercise, what these muscles are called, and how they affect posture. After the circuit, ask pupils to talk with a partner about the effects of the exercises on the musculoskeletal system (e.g., increases in muscular strength and endurance in specific muscle groups) and about how the muscle groups worked in the circuit help improve posture.

- Lead pupils through stretches for each of the muscle groups worked in the posture circuit—for example, prone or supine tummy stretch (station 1, rectus abdominis); seated, kneeling or standing cat stretch (station 2, erector spinae); backside stretch while lying on back with knees pulled towards chest (station 3, gluteus maximus); sides-of-tummy stretch while standing, seated or lying (station 4, obliques); and shoulder squeezes (station 5, trapezius). The stretching can be performed to calming background music.

- In the next lesson, following a warm-up (e.g., repeating the card game), add three more exercises to the posture circuit. For example, station 6 might involve push-ups (to address the pectorals and triceps), station 7 might involve squats (quadriceps and gluteus maximus), and station 8 might involve arm curls (biceps). As before, provide resource cards at the stations, showing visual images of up to three differentiated versions of each exercise. As before, the exercises can be performed for one minute at each station, and the circuit can be performed to background music.

- During the circuit, prompt pupils to think about which muscles are working in each exercise, what these muscles are called, and which everyday life activities and sporting activities benefit from improved strength and endurance in these muscle groups. After the circuit is completed, facilitate the sharing of responses with the class.

- Lead pupils through stretches for each of the muscle groups worked in the circuit. The stretches can be performed to calming background music.

ASSESSMENT OF HEALTH-RELATED LEARNING

- Towards the end of the unit of work, ask pupils questions such as the following:

- Why does your heart rate increase when you exercise?
- What happens to your breathing rate during energetic activity, and why?
- How does the body regulate its temperature during exercise?
- In what ways can your appearance change when you exercise, and why?
- Talk with a partner about exercises that you can do to improve your posture.

- Towards the end of the unit of work, involve pupils in active assessment tasks such as the following:

- Show me two exercises to develop tone in your abdominal muscles.
- Demonstrate how to develop the strength and endurance of your chest muscles.

HEALTH-RELATED LEARNING OUTCOMES: LESSONS 3 AND 4

ACTIVITY PROMOTION

- Explain that appropriate training can improve fitness and performance and that specific types of activity affect specific aspects of fitness (e.g., running affects cardiorespiratory fitness).

- Explain the differences between whole-body activities (e.g., walking, jogging, cycling, dancing, swimming) that help reduce body fat and conditioning exercises (e.g., straight and twisting curl-ups) that improve muscle tone.

HEALTH-RELATED LEARNING ACTIVITIES

- Involve pupils in a warm-up that gradually increases in intensity (e.g., working through the gears from first to fifth in the form of strolling, brisk walking, slow jogging, jogging and running) and includes a few static stretches of major muscle groups. Ask pupils to name the muscle groups being stretched.

- After the warm-up, ask pupils to talk in pairs or small groups about the effects of training. Prompt them to think about improvements

to fitness and performance. Facilitate sharing of their responses with the class.

- Involve pupils in an aerobic circuit—that is, a planned sequence of aerobic activities that develop cardiorespiratory fitness (e.g., skipping at station 1, knee lifts at station 2, squats at station 3, jogging at station 4 and sidesteps at station 5). Use resource cards for the stations. Exercises can be performed for one minute at each station, and the circuit can be performed to lively background music.

- After the aerobic circuit, ask pupils to talk with a partner about the effects of the exercises on the cardiorespiratory system (e.g., increases in stamina, cardiorespiratory fitness, ability to keep going for longer).

- Lead pupils through stretches for the major muscle groups worked in the aerobic circuit (e.g., quadriceps, calves, hamstrings, adductors, abductors). The stretching can be performed to calming background music.

- In the next lesson, expand the aerobic circuit by interspersing three exercises for muscular strength and endurance in the core muscles (e.g., curl-ups, back raises, twisting curl-ups). Involve pupils in the extended, eight-station circuit. Use resource cards showing visual images of differentiated versions of each exercise. The exercises can be performed for one minute at each station, and the circuit can be performed to background music.

- During the circuit, prompt pupils to think about which muscles are working in each exercise, what these muscles are called, and which everyday life activities and sporting activities benefit from improved strength and endurance in these muscle groups. After the circuit is completed, facilitate the sharing of responses with the class.
- Ask pupils to perform stretches for each of the muscle groups worked in the circuit.

The stretches can be performed to calming background music.

ASSESSMENT OF HEALTH-RELATED LEARNING

- Towards the end of the unit of work, involve pupils in active assessment tasks such as the following:
  - Match activities to components of fitness (e.g., running develops cardiorespiratory fitness).
  - Perform six whole-body activities; how do these activities help reduce body fat?
  - With a partner, perform four whole-body activities to music; put them into a sequence to teach to others.

HEALTH-RELATED LEARNING OUTCOMES: LESSONS 5 AND 6

HEALTH BENEFITS

- Explain a range of long-term benefits of activity for physical health, such as
  - reduced risk of chronic disease (e.g., heart disease),
  - reduced risk of bone disease (e.g., osteoporosis),
  - reduced risk of some other health conditions (e.g., obesity, back pain) and
  - improved management of some health conditions (e.g., asthma, diabetes, arthritis).
- Explain that activity can enhance mental health and social and psychological well-being (e.g., enjoyment of being with friends; increased confidence and self-esteem; decreased anxiety and stress) and that an appropriate balance between work, leisure and exercise promotes good health.
- Explain that increasing activity levels and eating a balanced diet can help one maintain a healthy body weight (i.e., energy balance), that the body needs a certain minimum daily energy intake in order to function properly and that strict dieting and excessive exercising can damage one's health.
- Explain how each activity area (athletics, dance, games, gymnastics, swimming and

outdoor and adventurous activities) can contribute to physical health and to social and psychological well-being (e.g., can improve stamina, assist in weight management, strengthen bones, be enjoyable).

HEALTH-RELATED LEARNING ACTIVITIES

- Ask pupils to talk in pairs or small groups about the long-term benefits of activity for physical health. Prompt them to consider reduced risk of some diseases and health conditions (e.g., heart disease, osteoporosis, obesity, back pain) and improved management of others (e.g., asthma, diabetes). Facilitate sharing of responses with the class.
- In small groups, ask pupils to choose six whole-body activities (e.g., walking, jogging, sidestepping, hopping, galloping) or movements (e.g., grapevines, high knee lifts, hopscotch). Then ask them to put these activities or movements into a sequence, set to music, that gradually increases in intensity (from low to moderate to vigorous). Pupils can then teach their sequence to others.
- Afterwards, ask pupils to walk with a partner or in their small group and talk about the mental and social health benefits of activity. Prompt them to consider benefits such as enjoyment of being with friends; increased self-confidence and self-esteem; and

decreased anxiety and stress. Afterwards, facilitate sharing of responses with the class.

- Lead pupils through a series of stretches set to calm, soothing music. Ask pupils how they feel afterwards (likely answers: relaxed, comfortable, good).

- In the next lesson, ask pupils what they know about energy balance—that is, the relationship between 'energy in' (i.e., taken in, in the form of calories from food and drink) and 'energy out' (i.e., used for everyday living, sleeping, activities and exercise) and the effect of this relationship on body weight. If energy in exceeds energy out, then body weight increases; if energy in and energy out are the same, then body weight remains the same; and if energy in is less than energy out, then body weight diminishes.

- To warm up, ask pupils to jog with a partner and chat about how activity can assist with healthy weight management. Afterwards, facilitate sharing of responses with the class.

- Ask pupils to participate in an energy balance game in which they select a food or drink card and perform sufficient activity to use up the calories listed for that food or drink—for example, for a chocolate biscuit (150 calories), 15 minutes of aerobic activity such as jogging or skipping. Use resource cards, each of which shows a visual image of a selected food or drink item, its calorie count, and activity choices for using up that number of calories. The game can be performed to background music.

- To finish the lesson, ask pupils to work in pairs or small groups to mime movements from a chosen activity area in a follow-my-leader fashion. Whilst doing so, they can talk about the health benefits of the activity area; for example, dance can improve stamina and flexibility, strengthen bones, assist with healthy weight management and be enjoyable.

ASSESSMENT OF HEALTH-RELATED LEARNING

- Towards the end of the unit of work, ask pupils questions such as the following:
  - How does being active help reduce your risk of heart disease?
  - How can activity help prevent you from getting bone conditions such as osteoporosis?
  - How does activity help individuals with asthma?
  - In what ways can activity help individuals feel good?
  - Name some activities that can calm or relax the body and mind.
  - Why is it important to balance work, leisure and exercise?
  - Explain to a partner what energy balance is.
  - Why is it essential to have a minimum daily energy intake?
  - How can strict dieting and excessive exercise affect your body and mind?
  - In a small group, match activity areas to health benefits (e.g., dance can improve stamina and flexibility, strengthen bones, assist with healthy weight management and be enjoyable).

- Towards the end of the unit of work, involve pupils in active assessment tasks such as the following:
  - Mime movements from an activity area and talk about health benefits of this area.
  - Jog with a partner and chat about how activity can assist with healthy weight management.

Short-term plans for health-related learning generally take the form of lesson plans with specific health-related learning outcomes that sit within units or blocks of work. The following example is a lesson plan for 12- and 13-year-olds that outlines learning outcomes for activity promotion within a health-related unit of work (focused on the physical activity recommendation and on keeping an activity diary), as well as learning activities to address the outcomes and suggested methods of assessing the learning.

HEALTH-RELATED LEARNING OUTCOMES

ACTIVITY PROMOTION

- Reflect on their activity strengths and preferences and know how to get involved in activities.
- Participate in activity of at least moderate intensity for one hour every day (accumulated over the course of a day), including activity that strengthens muscles and bones.
- Monitor and evaluate personal activity levels over a period of time (e.g., by keeping an activity diary for four to six weeks and reflecting on the experience).

HEALTH-RELATED LEARNING ACTIVITIES

- Ask pupils to discuss in pairs or small groups the types of activities and sports they like most and what they like about them. Then ask each pair or small group to share responses with another.
- Lead pupils through a series of whole-body aerobic activities such as the following examples. Start at low intensity and gradually shift to moderate intensity and then moderate-to-high intensity.
  - Strolling (low intensity)
  - Brisk walking (low to moderate)
  - Sidestepping (low to moderate)
  - Knee lifts (without jumps, low to moderate; with jumps, moderate to high)
  - Jogging (moderate to high)
  - Hopping (moderate to high)
  - Galloping (moderate to high)
  - Skipping (moderate to high)
- This series can be performed to lively background music. Afterwards, ask pupils to rate each of the activities from 1 to 10 in terms of how much they enjoyed performing them.
- Next, ask pupils how active children of their age should be. Then ask them to form pairs or small groups and look around in the area for cards (or sticky notes) stating how active young people should be. Each pair or group should collect three cards (in different colours, each colour representing part of the guideline) and place them together to form the complete guideline regarding physical activity for health for young people.
  - Guideline 1: All children and young people should engage in physical activity of moderate to vigorous intensity for at least 60 minutes and up to several hours every day.
  - Guideline 2: Vigorous-intensity activities, including those that strengthen muscle and bone, should be incorporated on at least three days per week.
  - Guideline 3: All children and young people should minimise the amount of time spent being sedentary for extended periods.
- Ask pupils to perform moderate-intensity activities; offer examples, such as knee raises, grapevines, squats and brisk walking. These activities can be performed to lively background music. Afterwards, ask pupils how they feel. Answers may include something like 'a little out of breath but comfortable' or 'able to keep going for a reasonable amount of time'.
- Now, ask pupils to perform moderate- to high-intensity activities; again, offer examples, such as knee raises with a jump, grapevines with a jump, deep squats and jogging. As before, the activities can be performed to lively background music. Afterwards, ask pupils how they feel. Answers may include something like 'out of breath' or 'unable to keep going for very long'.
- Assign pairs or small groups of pupils selected moderate-intensity activities (one each). Ask each pair or group to adapt its activity to vigorous intensity (e.g., by making the movements larger, deeper, quicker or higher). This activity can be performed to lively background music. Afterwards, pupils can share their ideas with the class, and class members can copy both the moderate version and the vigorous version presented by each group.
- Ask pupils to stretch large muscles used in whole-body aerobic activities, such as the quadriceps, hamstrings, calves, abductors and adductors. The stretching can be performed to calming background music.
- Introduce pupils to an activity diary and request that they use it for four weeks.

Ensure that pupils understand key terms such as *frequency, intensity* and *duration.* Ask pupils to write in today's activity so that they become familiar with the format and content of the diary. Remind them to bring their diary to each lesson in this unit of work. Inform them that in future lessons, they will be asked to reveal what their diary shows about their activity patterns and habits. For example, are they more active on weekdays or at weekends? Are they as active as they should be for their age?

ASSESSMENT OF HEALTH-RELATED LEARNING

- Towards the end of the unit of work, ask pupils questions such as the following:
  - Discuss your favourite activities and why you like them.
  - How much activity should young people do?
  - What does 'at least moderate intensity' mean?
  - Give me examples of activities that are of 'at least moderate intensity'.
  - Demonstrate moderate intensity and then vigorous intensity.
  - Explain to a partner what 'accumulated over the course of a day' means.

  - Keep an activity diary for four to six weeks; record all of the activity you do and its intensity and duration.

The web resource for this chapter provides a Gearing Up for Activity worksheet associated with the unit of work in which this lesson is located.

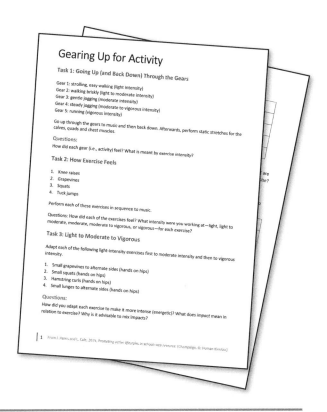

Gearing Up for Activity

Task 1: Going Up (and Back Down) Through the Gears

Gear 1: strolling, easy walking (light intensity)
Gear 2: walking briskly (light to moderate intensity)
Gear 3: gentle jogging (moderate intensity)
Gear 4: steady jogging (moderate to vigorous intensity)
Gear 5: running (vigorous intensity)

Go up through the gears to music and then back down. Afterwards, perform static stretches for the calves, quads and chest muscles.

Questions:
How did each gear (i.e., activity) feel? What is meant by exercise *intensity*?

Task 2: How Exercise Feels

1. Knee raises
2. Grapevines
3. Squats
4. Tuck jumps

Perform each of these exercises in sequence to music.

Questions: How did each of the exercises feel? What intensity were you working at—light, light to moderate, moderate, moderate to vigorous, or vigorous—for each exercise?

Task 3: Light to Moderate to Vigorous

Adapt each of the following light-intensity exercises first to moderate intensity and then to vigorous intensity.

1. Small grapevines to alternate sides (hands on hips)
2. Small squats (hands on hips)
3. Hamstring curls (hands on hips)
4. Small lunges to alternate sides (hands on hips)

Questions:
How did you adapt each exercise to make it more intense (energetic)? What does *impact* mean in relation to exercise? Why is it advisable to mix impacts?

1 From J. Harris and L. Cale, 2019, *Promoting active lifestyles in schools web resource* (Champaign, IL: Human Kinetics)

Summary

If you take a structured, progressive approach to children's learning about leading a healthy, active lifestyle, then you can engage them with this important aspect of the curriculum in a way that is comprehensive, coherent and meaningful. This sort of approach needs to be evident at all stages of schooling and be accessible to every pupil. A good way to start is to develop health-related learning plans that include relevant outcomes for successive age groups. The learning can then be organised, taught and assessed in multiple ways and can incorporate the monitoring of children's health, activity and fitness through methods that are developmentally appropriate and pedagogically desirable.

11

Health-Related Learning for 14- to 16-Year-Olds

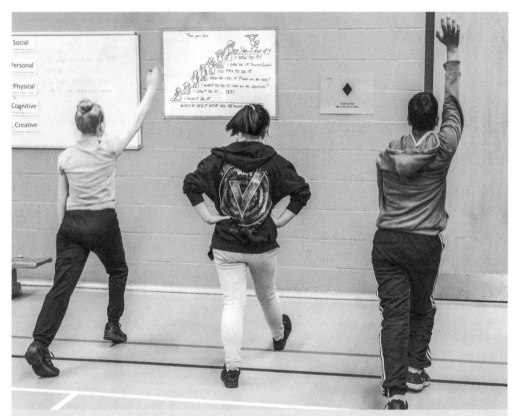

Chapter Objectives

After reading this chapter, you will be able to

- ▶ identify appropriate health-related learning outcomes and contexts for 14- to 16-year-olds;
- ▶ implement a variety of approaches to assess the health-related learning of 14- to 16-year-olds;
- ▶ describe methods of monitoring the health, activity and fitness of 14- to 16-year-olds; and
- ▶ create long-, medium- and short-term plans for health-related learning for 14- to 16-year-olds.

As with younger pupils, older secondary-school children need to learn about leading a healthy, active lifestyle in a manner that is structured, progressive and accessible to all pupils. The learning can be organised in multiple ways, including activity-based units of work in PE and separate health-related units in PE. This chapter proposes relevant health-related learning approaches for 14- to 16-year-olds and provides you with guidance for assessing pupils' learning. It also suggests methods for monitoring the health, activity and fitness of 14- to 16-year-olds, such as health behaviour questionnaires, activity diaries and questionnaires, heart rate monitors, pedometers and accelerometers, and developmentally appropriate fitness tests. Finally, the chapter provides sample schemes, units of work and lesson plans to help you create health-related learning plans that ensure a comprehensive, coherent and meaningful approach to this important aspect of the curriculum.

Health-Related Learning Outcomes and Contexts

As detailed in chapter 3, approaches to health-related learning for the 5- to 16-year-old age group were debated and agreed on in England in 2000 by a working group comprising representatives of national PE, sport and health organisations. Table 11.1 presents specific health-related learning outcomes for 14- to 16-year-olds; the outcomes are presented in four categories—safety issues, exercise effects, health benefits and activity promotion—to help clarify the scope and progression of the learning.

The learning content detailed in table 11.1 can be taught in a number of contexts. One approach is to integrate it into or permeate it through activity-based units of work in PE (e.g., athletics, dance, games, gymnastics, outdoor education and swimming lessons). Another approach is to teach it in separate thematic units of work in PE with a title such as Health-Related Exercise or Promoting Active Lifestyles. A third option is to combine the first two approaches. Limitations in these approaches (discussed in chapter 3) can be addressed by ensuring that learning outcomes integrated into or permeated through activity-based units of work in PE are not lost and do not take second place to other learning (e.g., skill development, tactical understanding,

choreography). In addition, learning outcomes taught in separate health-related units of work in PE should be connected closely with the rest of the PE curriculum and with the content and delivery of related subjects (e.g., science; food and technology; personal, social, health and economic [PSHE] education) and extracurricular and community activity experiences.

More specifically, the learning outcomes related to safety issues can be permeated through activity-based units of work in PE. The learning outcomes related to exercise effects and health benefits can be either permeated through activity-based units of work in PE or taught in additional health-related units of work. Explicit links should be made with PSHE education for this age group, which includes learning about where and how to obtain health information, advice and support and recognising and managing feelings about (and influences on) body image, including media portrayals of idealised and artificial body shapes (PSHE Association, 2014). The learning outcomes related to activity promotion can be either permeated through PE units of work or taught in additional health-related units of work. Here again, explicit links should be made with PSHE education for this age group, which in this case includes learning to take increased responsibility for monitoring one's own health (PSHE Association, 2014).

To ensure alignment with a whole-school approach to health, including the promotion of physical activity, information about activity opportunities on offer in the school and in the local community can be communicated to pupils and their families in a multitude of ways (e.g., via newsletters, posters, parent mail, parent consultations, assemblies). In addition, the school website can have a dedicated Where to Be Active section highlighting physical activity opportunities at school and within a five-mile radius of the school; this section can also be used to connect and support pupils (and families) involved in these activities.

Assessing Health-Related Learning

Health-related learning can be assessed via written, verbal and active responses to questions, tasks and tests. In terms of focus, assessment can address affective, behavioural or cognitive

TABLE 11.1 Health-Related Learning Outcomes for Ages 14 to 16

Pupils who are 14 to 16 years old can do the following:

Safety issues	• Recognise and manage risk and apply safe exercise principles and procedures (e.g., not exercising when unwell or injured; avoiding prolonged high-impact exercise; administering first aid, including resuscitation techniques; avoiding excessive amounts of exercise). • Evaluate warm-ups and cool-downs in terms of safety, effectiveness and relevance to the specific activity and take responsibility for their own safe and effective preparation for and recovery from activity. • Select, perform and evaluate exercises from a range of lifetime activities (e.g., jogging, swimming, cycling, aerobics, step aerobics, circuit training, weight training) with an eye toward safety, effectiveness and developmental appropriateness.
Exercise effects	• Explain that training exercises and practices affect performance and are activity specific. • Explain that training programmes develop both health-related components of physical and mental fitness (cardiorespiratory fitness, muscular strength and endurance, flexibility, body composition, composure and decision making) and skill-related components (agility, balance, coordination, power, reaction time, speed, concentration and determination).
Health benefits	• Explain that frequent and appropriate exercise enhances the physical, social and psychological well-being of all individuals, regardless of age, able-bodiedness or disability, and the presence or absence of health conditions (e.g., asthma, depression) and chronic disease (e.g., arthritis). • Explain that exercise can help one manage stress and contribute to a happy, healthy and balanced lifestyle. • Appreciate the risks associated with a sedentary lifestyle and with excessive behaviour (e.g., overexercising, disordered eating). • Identify how each activity area (e.g., gymnastics, swimming, athletics) can contribute to specific components of health-related fitness; for example, gymnastics involves weight-bearing actions and thus develops muscular strength and endurance.

Activity promotion	• Plan, perform, monitor and evaluate a safe and effective health-related exercise programme that meets their personal needs and preferences over an extended period of time (e.g., 6 to 12 weeks).
	• Access physical activity personnel (e.g., sport development officers, active school coordinators, coaches, instructors), facilities (e.g., leisure centres; sport, health and fitness clubs) and services (e.g., courses, projects, leaflets, pamphlets) in the local community.
	• Demonstrate a range of lifetime physical activities (e.g., walking, jogging, swimming, cycling, aerobics, step aerobics, circuit training, weight training, skipping, aqua exercise).
	• Explain and demonstrate practical understanding of the key principles of exercise programming and training, including
	  • progression (developing the amount of exercise by gradually increasing frequency, intensity, duration or a combination of these factors);
	  • overload (progressively enabling the body to do more exercise than accustomed to);
	  • specificity (doing a particular exercise or sporting activity to benefit specific muscles, joints, bones and energy systems);
	  • balance, moderation and variety (maximising exercise benefits and minimising risks);
	  • maintenance (establishing a routine, sustaining a commitment and coping with relapse);
	  • reversibility (gradually losing the benefits of exercise if it is discontinued); and
	  • cost–benefit ratio (weighing costs such as time, money, transport and sweat against benefits such as maintaining body weight, feeling good and improving health and fitness).
	• Assess their own qualities, skills, achievements and potential so that they can set personal goals that help them follow the activity recommendations for young people and develop a commitment to an active lifestyle.
	• Explain constraints on being active and explore how to overcome them in order to access and sustain involvement in activity.

(ABC) learning outcomes; for more on ABC outcomes, see chapter 3. Affective and behavioural outcomes for 14- to 16-year-olds can be assessed via teacher observation of effort and commitment in PE lessons, as well as participation records for PE lessons and extracurricular activities (using ratings such as excellent, good, satisfactory or adequate, and low or inadequate). Cognitive outcomes can be assessed through question-and-answer episodes and through practical and active tasks. Active assessment tasks are particularly encouraged because they increase activity levels in PE lessons (for more information about active assessment, see chapter 3). Table 11.2 presents a range of methods for assessing the recommended health-related learning outcomes for 14- to 16-year-olds.

TABLE 11.2   Methods of Assessing Health-Related Learning in 14- to 16-Year-Olds

Health-related learning category	Health-related learning outcomes	Methods of assessing health-related learning outcomes

Safety issues	• Recognise and manage risk and apply safe exercise principles and procedures (e.g., not exercising when unwell or injured; avoiding prolonged high-impact exercise; administering first aid, including resuscitation techniques; avoiding excessive amounts of exercise).
	• Evaluate warm-ups and cool-downs in terms of safety, effectiveness and relevance to the specific activity and take responsibility for their own safe and effective preparation for and recovery from activity.
	• Select, perform and evaluate exercises from a range of lifetime activities (e.g., jogging, swimming, cycling, aerobics, step aerobics, circuit training, weight training) with an eye toward safety, effectiveness and developmental appropriateness.
		• Ask pupils questions such as these:
		  • Why is it advisable to avoid exercise when you feel unwell or are injured?
		  • What are some possible effects of prolonged high-impact exercise?
		  • What would you do if a teammate bumped heads with an opponent and collapsed to the ground?
		  • Discuss with a partner what might be problematic about excessive exercising.
		  • What is involved in taking responsibility for your own safe and effective preparation for and recovery from activity?
		  • Observe a group's warm-up and provide feedback about its safety (e.g., occurs in an area cleared of potential hazards; intensity built up gradually), effectiveness (e.g., includes mobility exercises, aerobic activities and stretches) and relevance (relates to the activity to follow it).
		  • What does the term 'lifetime activity' mean?
		  • Name six lifetime activities.
		  • Which lifetime activities do you do? Could you do more?
		• Involve pupils in active assessment tasks such as these:
		  • Design and lead others through a warm-up for badminton that includes movements used in badminton and makes use of lines on a badminton court.
		  • In a small group, prepare yourselves for a 100-metre sprint.
		  • In a small group, plan and perform a cool-down to follow an 800-metre run.
		  • Demonstrate two lifetime activities.

Health-related learning category	Health-related learning outcomes	Methods of assessing health-related learning outcomes

Exercise effects	• Explain that training exercises and practices affect performance and are activity specific.
	• Explain that training programmes develop both health-related components of physical and mental fitness (cardiorespiratory fitness, muscular strength and endurance, flexibility, body composition, composure and decision making) and skill-related components (agility, balance, coordination, power, reaction time, speed, concentration and determination).
		• Ask pupils questions such as these:
		  • What sorts of exercises and practices would you expect to see in football training sessions? How and why might they differ from cricket training sessions?
		  • In what ways can training affect performance?
		  • Name the health-related components of fitness.
		  • Name two components of fitness associated with mental health.
		  • How is flexibility associated with health?
		  • Name the skill-related components of fitness.
		  • Talk with a partner about the differences between health-related and skill-related components of fitness.
		  • Which of the following components of fitness are health related: cardiorespiratory fitness, balance, body composition, power?
		  • Which two of the following components of fitness are skill related: agility, muscular strength and endurance, flexibility, reaction time?
		• Involve pupils in active assessment tasks such as these:
		  • Mime each of the skill-related components of fitness.
		  • Pair up and take turns acting out a health-related or skill-related component of fitness while your partner guesses the component.

Health benefits	• Explain that frequent and appropriate exercise enhances the physical, social and psychological well-being of all individuals, regardless of age, able-bodiedness or disability, and the presence or absence of health conditions (e.g., asthma, depression) and chronic disease (e.g., arthritis).
	• Explain that exercise can help one manage stress and contribute to a happy, healthy and balanced lifestyle.
	• Appreciate the risks associated with a sedentary lifestyle and with excessive behaviour (e.g., overexercising, disordered eating).
	• Identify how each activity area (e.g., gymnastics, swimming, athletics) can contribute to specific components of health-related fitness; for example, gymnastics involves weight-bearing actions and thus develops muscular strength and endurance.
		• Ask pupils questions such as these:
		  • What are the physical benefits of physical activity?
		  • Talk with a partner about the social benefits of being active.
		  • How can physical activity benefit psychological well-being?
		  • Is physical activity beneficial to people of all ages? Support your answer with examples.
		  • Name some activities that can help one manage stress and anxiety.
		  • What are the risks of a sedentary lifestyle?
		  • How might overexercising be a problem?
		  • In a small group, match components of health-related fitness to relevant activity areas.
		  • Which activity area contributes most to cardiorespiratory fitness?
		• Involve pupils in active assessment tasks such as the following:
		  • Jog with a partner and chat about how being active can assist in healthy weight management.
		  • Walk briskly in a pair or small group and discuss how regular physical activity can help to reduce stress.

(continued)

Table 11.2 *(continued)*

Health-related learning category	Health-related learning outcomes	Methods of assessing health-related learning outcomes

Activity promotion	• Plan, perform, monitor and evaluate a safe and effective health-related exercise programme that meets their personal needs and preferences over an extended period of time (e.g., 6 to 12 weeks).
	• Access physical activity personnel (e.g., sport development officers, active school coordinators, coaches, instructors), facilities (e.g., leisure centres; sport, health and fitness clubs) and services (e.g., courses, projects, leaflets, pamphlets) in the local community.
	• Demonstrate a range of lifetime physical activities (e.g., walking, jogging, swimming, cycling, aerobics, step aerobics, circuit training, weight training, skipping, aqua exercise).
	• Explain and demonstrate practical understanding of the key principles of exercise programming and training, including
	  • progression (developing the amount of exercise by gradually increasing frequency, intensity, duration or a combination of these factors);
	  • overload (progressively enabling the body to do more exercise than accustomed to);
	  • specificity (doing a particular exercise or sporting activity to benefit specific muscles, joints, bones and energy systems);
	  • balance, moderation and variety (maximising exercise benefits and minimising risks);
	  • maintenance (establishing a routine, sustaining a commitment and coping with relapse);
	  • reversibility (gradually losing the benefits of exercise if it is discontinued); and
	  • cost–benefit ratio (weighing costs such as time, money, transport and sweat against benefits such as maintaining body weight, feeling good and improving health and fitness).
	• Assess their own qualities, skills, achievements and potential so that they can set personal goals that help them follow the activity recommendations for young people and develop a commitment to an active lifestyle.
	• Explain constraints on being active and explore how to overcome them in order to access and sustain involvement in activity.
		• Ask pupils questions such as these:
		  • What activities do you enjoy doing?
		  • What are your activity needs?
		  • Discuss with a partner the various sources of information available about activity opportunities in the local community.
		  • What makes lifetime activities beneficial?
		  • How can you achieve progression in an exercise programme?
		  • What does *overload* mean in relation to exercise?
		  • Discuss with a partner what *specificity* means and share some examples with the class.
		  • Why are balance, moderation and variety important when planning an exercise programme?
		  • What helps people maintain an exercise programme?
		  • What does *reversibility* mean in relation to exercise?
		  • With a partner, weigh up the costs and benefits of following a three-month exercise programme.
		  • Set personal activity goals, taking into consideration your current activity levels, abilities and preferences.
		• Involve pupils in active assessment tasks such as these:
		  • Show me where you can find information about activity opportunities in the local community.
		  • Walk and jog with a partner while talking about barriers and constraints related to being active and how to overcome them.
		  • Plan, perform, monitor and evaluate a safe and effective health-related exercise programme for a school term that meets your personal needs and preferences.

Monitoring Health, Activity and Fitness

The rationale for monitoring children's health, activity and fitness has been strengthened in recent years both by increased concern about children's physical, mental and social health and by the trend towards sedentary living that marks a more technologically advanced world. These issues are addressed in part I of this book, whereas part II covers developmentally and pedagogically appropriate approaches to monitoring within the curriculum in order to promote healthy, active lifestyles among children. The following examples are appropriate for use with 14- to 16-year-olds.

Monitoring Health

We can help children become more aware of their lifestyles by using health behaviour questionnaires that offer a selection of responses (e.g., always, mostly, sometimes, never) to questions such as the following:

- Do you drink about six glasses of water per day?
- Do you get enough sleep (about 8 to 10 hours per night)?
- Do you usually remain in control of your emotions?
- Can you adequately cope with the day-to-day pressures and stresses of your work and personal life?
- Are you active for about an hour every day?

Chapter 4 provides an example of a health behaviour questionnaire suitable for secondary-age pupils; it can be used to calculate a health score linked to generic feedback such as the following: 'Oh dear, it seems that you lead an unhealthy lifestyle and are likely to suffer the consequences, now and in the future. You should consider choosing a much healthier lifestyle by improving on many of your habits'. Engaging children in the process of self-reflection enhances learning and helps children to set measurable targets for improvement. Here are a few sample questions to ask 14- to 16-year-olds: 'What does your overall health score tell you? Are there parts of your health that you cannot change? If yes, which parts are they, and what is stopping you from changing them? On a scale of 0 to 10, how confident are you that you will be able to improve your health over the next three months?' Additional examples of self-reflection questions are provided in chapter 4.

Responses to these questions can be used to trigger discussions among pupils about ways to lead a healthy lifestyle, as well as relevant barriers and facilitators. Pupils aged 14 to 16 could also be involved in reviewing case study examples of young people's lifestyles (available for printing from the web resource for chapter 4) and considering answers to the following questions:

- How healthy is this person?
- What, if anything, could this person do to improve his or her health?

- What might help the person do so?
- What might prevent him or her from doing so?

Pupils could also be encouraged to write a short narrative, profile or blog paragraph about their own lifestyle. These responses could be used anonymously to discuss what it means to be healthy, how health is affected by factors both within and beyond an individual's control and what can be done both collectively and individually to improve public health.

When conducting such discussions, be sensitive to the fact that children of all ages (including older secondary-age children) have no control over major factors that influence their health—for example, genetics, environment (e.g., pollution, poverty) and family modelling. In addition, they have only partial control over other key factors, including what they eat and drink and how active they are. So, whilst children can learn about leading a healthy lifestyle (and the consequences of not doing so), they should also be aware of which factors influencing their health lie beyond their control and which ones they have some control over. Furthermore, leading a healthy lifestyle can cost more in terms of purchasing healthy foods and drinks and accessing physical activity opportunities (e.g., after-school or holiday clubs) that require payment. As a consequence, children from low-income families may be disadvantaged in comparison with their peers and, where possible, should be offered free or low-cost opportunities to consume healthy meals and drinks and to be active.

Monitoring Activity

As described in chapter 5, children's physical activity can be monitored through a number of methods. One appropriate method for 14- to 16-year-olds involves self-reporting—for example, keeping a physical activity diary for as long as a school term (for examples of activity diaries suitable for this age group, see the web resource for chapter 5). More-formal self-report instruments suitable for use with secondary-age children include the Previous Day Physical Activity Recall (PDPAR), the Three-Day Physical Activity Recall (3DPAR), the Physical Activity Questionnaire for Children (PAQ-C) or for Adolescents (PAQ-A), the Youth Risk Behaviour Surveillance System (YRBSS) and the Teen Health Survey. For more information about these instruments, see Trost (2007) and Biddle, Gorely, Pearson, & Bull (2011). Additional methods suitable for

14- to 16-year-olds include the use of pedometers, accelerometers and heart rate monitors (i.e., chest-strap transmitters paired with a wrist receiver or mobile phone); for a discussion of the advantages and disadvantages of these methods, see chapter 5. In recent years, accelerometers have also been developed into popular wearable electronic devices (e.g., Fitbit) that monitor physical activity and provide additional information and feedback on specific aspects of activity.

You can encourage pupils to reflect on their activity levels by asking questions such as the following: Do you usually take part in some moderate to vigorous activity each day? Are you active enough for your age? On a scale of 0 to 5, how motivated do you feel to be more active over the next month? (For more examples appropriate for secondary-age children, see the web resource for chapter 5).

You may also want to incorporate questions about sedentary behaviour into discussions about healthy lifestyles. This approach links with the UK-wide physical activity guideline that children and young people should minimise the amount of time spent being sedentary (for more information about this and other guidelines, see chapter 1). Young people's responses to questions such as 'When and where are you sedentary for extended periods of time?' and 'In what ways could this sedentary time be reduced or broken up?' can be used to promote discussion about the consequences of prolonged sedentary behaviour, as well as ways in which the school and local environments could encourage less sedentary behaviour.

Whilst obtaining a precise measure of physical activity is important for research purposes, it is less crucial for teachers, whose main concerns relate to the educational value of the monitoring experience and its ease of use, feasibility and cost. From a pedagogical perspective, it is considered more important to ensure that pupils enjoy, learn and benefit from the monitoring experience

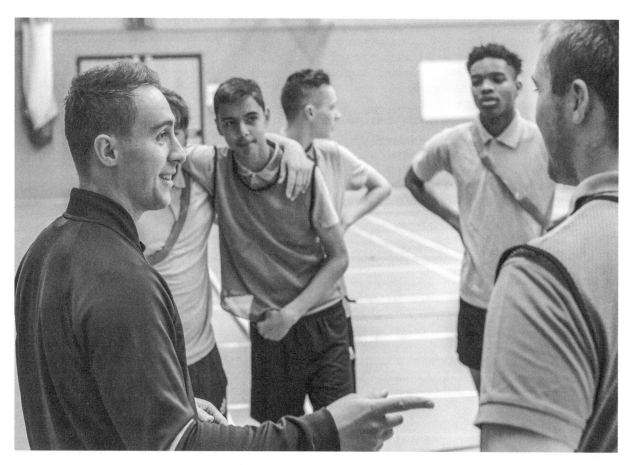

Teachers can help older secondary school children to appreciate the benefits of and to adopt healthy, active lifestyles.

than to worry unduly about the precision of the method (Cale & Harris, 2009b). This learning can include knowing how to incorporate physical activity into their lifestyles, knowing how to get involved in organised activities and reflecting on their activity strengths and preferences.

Pupils should be encouraged to think of ways in which they could be more physically active at school, at home and in the local community. Their responses can be used to prompt discussion about healthy, active lifestyles, including consideration of what helps and what hinders their participation in physical activity. Pupils can also be encouraged to discuss and critique visual images in the media in order to challenge common misunderstandings and misconceptions about physical activity—for example, believing that routine, habitual activities (e.g., walking to school or the shops) provide no health benefits and that competitive sport offers the greatest health benefits (see chapter 1 for a discussion of young people's inaccurate and inadequate understandings of health, fitness and physical activity).

Monitoring Fitness

As discussed in chapter 6, fitness testing is controversial in a school setting, and before using it with children we must consider a number of issues and limitations. Fitness monitoring can be considered a valuable component of the curriculum if it is developmentally appropriate; offers a positive, educational experience for all learners; and helps promote healthy, active lifestyles (Association for Physical Education, 2015a, 2015b; Cale, 2016; Cale & Harris, 2009a, 2009b; Cale, Harris, & Chen, 2014; Lloyd, Colley, & Tremblay, 2010; Rowland, 2007; Silverman, Keating, & Phillips, 2008).

It is not essential for children aged 14 to 16 to be involved in formal fitness testing in order for them to learn that certain activities develop fitness (e.g., aerobics improves cardiorespiratory fitness; back raises and twisting curl-ups improve strength and endurance in specific muscle groups). These associations can be taught in PE lessons, where children learn, for example, that aqua aerobics and table tennis help improve their cardiorespiratory fitness, flexibility and muscular strength and endurance.

If you choose to involve 14- to 16-year-olds in formal fitness testing, select the tests carefully and teach them in a positive, supportive setting.

Emphasise helping pupils enjoy and learn from the experience and strive to improve on their own personal-best scores. Submaximal tests are recommended for this age group—for example, the step test and the mini bleep test for cardiorespiratory fitness and differentiated versions of exercises for muscular strength and endurance (e.g., curl-up, push-up). The web resource for chapter 6 provides descriptions of these tests, as well as recommendations to consider before, during and after implementing them. Once fitness testing is complete, ask pupils to reflect on the experience and on their scores. The web resource for chapter 6 provides examples of appropriate questions for secondary-age children, such as the following: How do you feel about your scores? Were they as you expected, or were there any surprises? Are there areas of fitness where you feel you need to improve? If so, which ones? What are your views about fitness monitoring? Are there pros and cons?

All children aged 14 to 16 years should be helped to understand that fitness is developed by being physically active and is associated with good health. This message is consistent with the goal of influencing the process (being active) rather than the product (fitness) (Cale & Harris, 2009b). In addition, pupils can be encouraged to discuss and critique images from the media relating to fitness in order to challenge any misunderstandings and misconceptions that they may have about fitness—for example, believing that one must be good at sport in order to be fit or that fitness is about being thin (see chapter 1 for a discussion of young people's inaccurate and inadequate understandings of health, fitness and physical activity).

Health-Related Learning Plans for 14- to 16-Year-Olds

Long-term health-related plans generally take the form of a scheme of work over a number of years. In the case of 14- to 16-year-olds, the duration of the scheme of work is two academic years. Ideally, the health-related learning should sit within a whole-school approach to the promotion of health (see chapter 2) and can be taught within a number of contexts—for example, integrating it into activity-based units of work in PE and into separate, thematic health-related units of work in

LINKING CURRICULUM AND COMMUNITY

A secondary school in the Midlands undertook a review of its PE provision for older pupils. Teachers were keen to ensure that the PE curriculum for 14- to 16-year-olds helped pupils make links with activity opportunities in the community in order to increase the proportion choosing to be active, both in their own time whilst at school and outside of school. As part of this process, teachers undertook focus group discussions with pupils in order to take into consideration their views. Following the review, in the first few lessons of the autumn term, 14-year-old pupils were given activity journals to maintain throughout the next two years. They were guided to record short-, medium- and long-term personal activity goals and select activities for each term of the two-year period to help them meet their goals.

> **Discussion points:** What are the advantages of ensuring close links between curriculum and community opportunities for older pupils? What types of short-, medium- and long-term physical activity goals are appropriate for this age range?

The range of activities on offer involved making good use of nearby leisure and sport facilities, including a dance school, a swimming pool, a golf course, a horse-riding school and a bowling green. The activities were co-delivered by teachers and trained coaches and activity instructors. In order to increase the range of activities offered, a number of non-PE teachers with coaching qualifications were also involved. Personnel at the external activity venues provided pupils with information (i.e., brochures, leaflets) about how to join existing activities, and some gave presentations to pupils during the two-year period.

> **Discussion points:** Why do you think the activities were co-delivered by teachers and trained coaches and activity instructors? What are the potential benefits of this type of programme for schools and for the external agencies involved? What drawbacks or limitations might there be?

Towards the end of the programme's second year, focus group discussions were conducted with pupils to ascertain their views on the PE provision they had received. The pupils were generally positive about the changes and the increased range of opportunities. Many had used community facilities during the programme of which they had previously been unaware, and some had used these facilities outside of school time.

At the same time, a number of issues were identified, including relatively low uptake and monitoring of the activity journals over the two years, as well as too few places being available in some activities that were particularly popular. In addition, the costs of activities varied, and staff concluded that increased funding was needed to support the continuation of more expensive activities (e.g., golf, horse riding). They also decided that involving more non-PE staff would increase the appeal of the programme by extending the opportunities on offer. Finally, they decided to make a case to the school governors for funding to support the development of the programme, including the costs of coaching courses for non-PE staff who were keen to further develop a sporting hobby or interest and obtain a coaching qualification.

> **Discussion points:** What might be the reasons for the relatively low uptake and monitoring of the activity journals? Is this aspect of the programme worth developing further? Why, or why not? If so, how might it be developed? What are your views on increasing the involvement of non-PE teachers in curriculum PE provision?

PE. Learning outcomes that are integrated into or permeated through activity-based units of work in PE should not be lost or allowed to take second place to other learning (e.g., skill development, tactical understanding, choreography), and outcomes addressed through separate health-related units of work in PE should relate closely to the rest of the PE curriculum and to the content and delivery of related subjects (e.g., science, food technology, PSHE education).

Sample Health-Related Scheme of Work for 11- to 14-Year-Olds

The health-related learning identified in this example spans two academic years and is taught through activity-based units of work in PE in combination with separate, thematic health-related units of work in PE called Promoting Active Lifestyles (PAL). This learning sits within a whole-school approach to health that aims to achieve healthy lifestyles for the entire school population by developing a supportive environment that is conducive to promoting health through the curriculum, the environment and the community.

HEALTH-RELATED LEARNING CATEGORY: SAFETY ISSUES

HEALTH-RELATED LEARNING OUTCOMES

- Recognise and manage risk and apply safe exercise principles and procedures (e.g., not exercising when unwell or injured; avoiding prolonged high-impact exercise; administering first aid, including resuscitation techniques; avoiding excessive amounts of exercise).
- Evaluate warm-ups and cool-downs in terms of safety, effectiveness and relevance to the specific activity and take responsibility for their own safe and effective preparation for and recovery from activity
- Select, perform and evaluate exercises from a range of lifetime activities (e.g., jogging, swimming, cycling, aerobics, step aerobics, circuit training, weight training) with an eye toward safety, effectiveness and developmental appropriateness.

HEALTH-RELATED LEARNING CONTEXT

These learning outcomes are taught in activity-based units of work in curriculum PE with explicit links to safety issues that arise within extracurricular and community settings (e.g., applying safe exercise principles and procedures, taking responsibility for safe and effective preparation for and recovery from activity, performing lifetime activities).

METHODS OF ASSESSING HEALTH-RELATED LEARNING OUTCOMES

Ask pupils questions such as the following:

- Why is it best to avoid exercise when you feel unwell or are injured?
- What are some possible effects of prolonged high-impact exercise?
- What would you do if a teammate bumped heads with an opponent and collapsed to the ground?
- Discuss with a partner what might be problematic about excessive exercising.
- What is involved in taking responsibility for your own safe and effective preparation for and recovery from activity?
- Observe a group's warm-up and provide feedback about its safety (e.g., occurs in an area cleared of potential hazards; builds intensity gradually), effectiveness (includes mobility exercises, aerobic activities and stretches) and relevance (relates to the activity to follow it).
- What does the term 'lifetime activity' mean?
- Name six lifetime activities.
- Which lifetime activities do you do? Could you do more?

Involve pupils in active assessment tasks such as the following:

- Design and lead others through a warm-up for badminton that includes movements used in badminton and makes use of lines on a badminton court.
- In a small group, prepare for a 100-metre sprint.
- In a small group, plan and perform a cool-down to follow an 800-metre run.
- Demonstrate two lifetime activities.

HEALTH-RELATED LEARNING CATEGORY: EXERCISE EFFECTS

HEALTH-RELATED LEARNING OUTCOMES

- Explain that training exercises and practices affect performance and are activity specific.
- Explain that training programmes develop both health-related components of physical and mental fitness (cardiorespiratory fitness, muscular strength and endurance, flexibility, body composition, composure and decision making) and skill-related components (agility, balance, coordination, power, reaction time, speed, concentration and determination).

HEALTH-RELATED LEARNING CONTEXT

These learning outcomes are taught in activity-based and health-related units of work in curriculum PE with explicit links to related learning in PSHE, science and food technology.

METHODS OF ASSESSING HEALTH-RELATED LEARNING OUTCOMES

Ask pupils questions such as the following:

- What sorts of exercises and practices would you expect to see in football training sessions? How and why might they differ from cricket training sessions?

- In what ways can training affect performance?
- Name the health-related components of fitness.
- Name two components of fitness associated with mental health.
- How is flexibility associated with health?
- Name the skill-related components of fitness.
- Talk with a partner about the differences between health-related and skill-related components of fitness.
- Which of the following components of fitness are health related: cardiorespiratory fitness, balance, body composition, power?
- Which two of the following components of fitness are skill related: agility, muscular strength and endurance, flexibility, reaction time?

Involve pupils in active assessment tasks such as the following:

- Mime each of the skill-related components of fitness.
- Pair up and take turns acting out a health-related or skill-related component of fitness while your partner guesses the component.

HEALTH-RELATED LEARNING CATEGORY: HEALTH BENEFITS

HEALTH-RELATED LEARNING OUTCOMES

- Explain that frequent and appropriate exercise enhances the physical, social and psychological well-being of all individuals, regardless of age, able-bodiedness or disability, and the presence or absence of health conditions (e.g., asthma, depression) and chronic disease (e.g., arthritis).
- Explain that exercise can help one manage stress and contribute to a happy, healthy and balanced lifestyle.

- Appreciate the risks associated with a sedentary lifestyle and with excessive behaviour (e.g., overexercising, disordered eating).
- Identify how each activity area (e.g., gymnastics, swimming, athletics) can contribute to specific components of health-related fitness; for example, gymnastics involves weight-bearing actions and thus develops muscular strength and endurance.

HEALTH-RELATED LEARNING CONTEXT

These learning outcomes are taught in health-related units of work in PE called Promoting Active Lifestyles (PAL) with explicit links to learning in activity-based units of work in PE and in PSHE.

METHODS OF ASSESSING HEALTH-RELATED LEARNING OUTCOMES

Ask pupils questions such as the following:

- What are the physical benefits of physical activity?
- Talk with a partner about the social benefits of being active.
- How can physical activity benefit psychological well-being?
- Is physical activity beneficial to people of all ages? Support your answer with examples.

- Name some activities that can help one manage stress and anxiety.
- What are the risks of a sedentary lifestyle?
- How might overexercising be a problem?
- In a small group, match components of health-related fitness to each activity area.
- Which activity area contributes most to cardiorespiratory fitness?

Involve pupils in active assessment tasks such as the following:

- Jog with a partner while chatting about how being active can assist with healthy weight management.
- Walk briskly in a pair or small group and discuss how activity can help people to feel better about themselves.

HEALTH-RELATED LEARNING CATEGORY: ACTIVITY PROMOTION

HEALTH-RELATED LEARNING OUTCOMES

- Plan, perform, monitor and evaluate a safe and effective health-related exercise programme that meets their personal needs and preferences over an extended period of time (e.g., 6 to 12 weeks).
- Access physical activity personnel (e.g., sport development officers, active school coordinators, coaches, instructors), facilities (e.g., leisure centres; sport, health and fitness clubs) and services (e.g., courses, projects, leaflets, pamphlets) in the local community.
- Demonstrate a range of lifetime physical activities (e.g., walking, jogging, swimming, cycling, aerobics, step aerobics, circuit training, weight training, skipping, aqua exercise).
- Explain and demonstrate practical understanding of the key principles of exercise programming and training, including
  - progression (developing the amount of exercise by gradually increasing fre-

quency, intensity, duration or a combination of these factors);
  - overload (progressively enabling the body to do more exercise than accustomed to);
  - specificity (doing a particular exercise or sporting activity to benefit specific muscles, joints, bones and energy systems);
  - balance, moderation and variety (maximising exercise benefits and minimising risks);
  - maintenance (establishing a routine, sustaining a commitment and coping with relapse);
  - reversibility (gradually losing the benefits of exercise if it is discontinued); and
  - cost–benefit ratio (weighing costs such as time, money, transport and sweat against benefits such as maintaining body weight, feeling good and improving health and fitness).
- Assess their own qualities, skills, achievements and potential so that they can set personal goals that help them follow the

activity recommendations for young people and develop a commitment to an active lifestyle.

- Explain constraints on being active and explore how to overcome them in order to access and sustain involvement in activity.

HEALTH-RELATED LEARNING CONTEXT

These learning outcomes are taught in health-related units of work in PE called Promoting Active Lifestyles (PAL) with explicit links to learning in activity-based units of work in PE and in PSHE.

METHODS OF ASSESSING HEALTH-RELATED LEARNING OUTCOMES

Ask questions such as the following:

- What activities do you enjoy doing?
- What are your activity needs?
- Discuss with a partner the sources of information available about activity opportunities in the local community.
- What makes lifetime activities beneficial?
- How can you achieve progression in an exercise programme?
- What does *overload* mean in relation to exercise?

- Discuss with a partner what *specificity* means in relation to exercise and think of some examples to share with the class.
- Why are balance, moderation and variety important when planning an exercise programme?
- What helps people maintain an exercise programme?
- What does *reversibility* mean in relation to exercise?
- With a partner, weigh up the costs and benefits of following a three-month exercise programme.
- Set personal activity goals, taking into consideration your current activity levels, abilities and preferences.

Involve pupils in active assessment tasks such as the following:

- Show me where you can find information about activity opportunities in the local community.
- Walk and jog with a partner while talking about barriers and constraints related to being active and how to overcome them.
- Plan, perform, monitor and evaluate a safe and effective health-related exercise programme for a school term that meets your personal needs and preferences.

Medium-term plans for health-related learning generally take the form of units of work over the course a school term (usually 10 to 14 weekly lessons) or parts of a term (usually 4 to 7 weekly lessons). These units of work are likely to be within the subject of PE (activity based and health related) with explicit links to learning in related subjects such as PSHE education, science and food technology.

Sample Health-Related Unit of Work for 14- to 16-Year-Olds

The following example presents a six-lesson, topic-based unit called Promoting Active Lifestyles (PAL) and outlines selected learning outcomes for activity promotion for 14- and 15-year-olds. It also covers learning activities to address the outcomes, as well as suggested methods for assessing pupils' learning. The learning in this unit is cross-referenced to related learning in activity-based units of work in PE.

HEALTH-RELATED LEARNING OUTCOMES: LESSONS 1 AND 2

ACTIVITY PROMOTION

- Plan, perform, monitor and evaluate a safe and effective health-related exercise programme that meets personal needs and preferences over an extended period of time (e.g., 6 to 12 weeks).

- Access physical activity personnel (e.g., sport development officers, active school coordinators, coaches, instructors), facilities (e.g., leisure centres; sport, health and fitness clubs) and services (e.g., courses, projects, leaflets, pamphlets) in the local community.

- Demonstrate a range of lifetime physical activities (e.g., walking, jogging, swimming, cycling, aerobics, step aerobics, circuit training, weight training, skipping, aqua exercise).

HEALTH-RELATED LEARNING ACTIVITIES

- Lead pupils through a task in which they perform exercises of increasing intensity (e.g., alternate knee raises without a jump, grapevines without a jump, squats and tuck jumps). After each exercise, ask pupils to describe its intensity as either easy (low or light intensity), comfortable (low or light intensity to moderate intensity), a little hard (moderate intensity), very hard (moderate to high or vigorous intensity), or exhausting (high or vigorous intensity).

- During the activity, ask the following: What does intensity mean? Are the descriptions the same for each exercise? Why is this?

- Ask pupils to complete the following progressive tasks on the Cardio Activity Task sheet found in the web resource:
  - Impact circuit
  - Impact and intensity circuit

- Afterwards, ask pupils to perform stretches for the major muscle groups in the impact and intensity circuit.

- Towards the end of the first lesson, provide pupils with an activity journal that guides them in designing an activity programme that meets their personal needs and preferences. Ask them to plan and maintain their activity programme for a school term and to record the frequency, duration and intensity of the activity they do at school, at home

and in the community. Check that pupils know where to find information about activity opportunities in the community, including whom to ask. Encourage them to make sure that their programme includes habitual, routine and lifetime activities.

- In the next lesson, ask pupils to work in pairs or small groups to complete the Everyday Activities Task found in the web resource. This task guides them in designing and

Cardio Activity Task

Impact Circuit

Design a moderate to vigorous intensity aerobic activity for each task in the table.

Task	Impact	Instruction
1	High	
2	Low	Travelling around the area
3	High	Side to side
4	Low	On the spot
		Forwards and backwards

Questions:
How did you know that the activities you designed were moderate to vigorous activity? What are the benefits of weight-bearing activity? What are the possible risks of excessive high impact exercise?

Impact and Intensity Circuit

Design exercises that answer each task in the table. Perform each exercise to music for about one minute and then move straight on to the next task.

Task	Impact	Intensity	Instruction
1	Low	Moderate	Side to side
2	High	Moderate	Travelling
3	Low	Vigorous	On the spot
4	High	Moderate	With a kick
5	Low	Vigorous	With a clap
6	High	Moderate	Forward and backward
7	Low	Vigorous	Change of direction
8	High	Moderate	In a small circle

1   From J. Harris and L. Cale, 2019, *Promoting active lifestyles in schools web resource.* (Champaign, IL: Human Kinetics).

Everyday Activities Task

The table below lists some everyday activities (1st column) and the location of the main muscles used in these (2nd column). Think of an appropriate resistance exercise for each muscle location listed in column 2 and write its name in column 4.

Perform a circuit containing these 8 exercises. Before you start, look at the exercise target (final column) and decide your own starting point for building up to this. After each exercise, record how it felt (in column 5 - see scale below).

Everyday activity	Location of muscles working	Number of exercise station	Exercise name	How the exercise feels	Starting point	Exercise target
Standing (which muscles support the spine and head?)	Along length of tummy	1				
	Along length of spine	2				8-12 reps (hard) twice per week
	Sides of tummy	3				
	Across shoulders	4				
Climbing stairs, sitting down and getting up	Front of upper leg	5				
	Backside	6				8-12 reps (hard) twice per week
Lifting and lowering a heavy bag or pulling with arms	Front of upper arm	7				8-12 reps (hard) twice per week
Pushing with arms	Back of upper arm	8				8-12 reps (hard) twice per week

How the exercise feels
Easy
Comfortable
Hard
Very Hard
Exhausting

Question
What happens if muscles we use every day start to tire easily?

1   From J. Harris and L. Cale, 2019, *Promoting active lifestyles in schools web resource.* (Champaign, IL: Human Kinetics).

performing a circuit of exercises to tone and strengthen the major muscle groups involved in everyday activities (e.g., standing; climbing stairs; sitting down; getting up; and lifting, lowering, pulling and pushing objects).

- During the circuit, ask pupils to think about how toning and strengthening these muscle groups assists with everyday activities.
- Ask pupils to perform stretches for the major muscle groups used in the everyday activities circuit.

ASSESSMENT OF HEALTH-RELATED LEARNING

- Towards the end of the unit of work, ask pupils questions such as the following:

  - What activities do you enjoy doing?
  - What are your activity needs?
  - Discuss with a partner the sources of information available about activity opportunities in the local community.
  - What makes lifetime activities beneficial?

- Towards the end of the unit of work, involve pupils in active assessment tasks such as the following:

  - Show me where you can find information about activity opportunities in the local community.
  - Plan, perform, monitor and evaluate a safe and effective health-related exercise programme for a school term that meets your personal needs and preferences.

HEALTH-RELATED LEARNING OUTCOMES: LESSONS 3 AND 4

ACTIVITY PROMOTION

- Explain and demonstrate practical understanding of the key principles of exercise programming and training, including

  - progression (developing the amount of exercise by gradually increasing frequency, intensity, duration or a combination of these factors);
  - overload (progressively enabling the body to do more exercise than accustomed to);
  - specificity (doing a particular exercise or sporting activity to benefit specific muscles, joints, bones and energy systems);
  - balance, moderation and variety (maximising exercise benefits and minimising risks);
  - maintenance (establishing a routine, sustaining a commitment and coping with relapse);
  - reversibility (gradually losing the benefits of exercise if it is discontinued); and
  - cost–benefit ratio (weighing costs such as time, money, transport and sweat against benefits such as maintaining body weight, feeling good and improving health and fitness).

HEALTH-RELATED LEARNING ACTIVITIES

- Ask pupils to work in pairs or small groups to match key principles of exercise programming and training written on a set of cards (e.g., progression, overload, specificity, reversibility, maintenance) with their descriptions written on a different set of cards. Afterwards, ask questions to check pupils' understanding of these terms and how the principles can be applied when designing exercise and training programmes.
- Ask pupils to work in pairs or small groups to complete a sport performance task. The task should guide them to design and perform a circuit of exercises to strengthen the major muscle groups used in basketball actions (e.g., jumping high, lunging and dodging from side to side, sprinting, jogging, throwing, shooting, travelling).
- During the sport performance circuit, ask pupils to think about how strengthening these muscle groups can help improve their performance in basketball.
- Ask pupils to perform stretches for the major muscle groups used in basketball.

- In the next lesson, ask pupils to work in pairs or small groups to design and perform a circuit of exercises to strengthen the major muscle groups involved in an activity or sport of their choice.

- During the circuit, ask pupils to think about how strengthening these muscle groups can help improve their performance in their selected activity or sport.

- Ask pupils to perform stretches for the major muscle groups used in their selected activity or sport.

- Ask pupils to consider the importance of balance, moderation and variety in exercise and training programmes and the cost–benefit ratio of activity or exercise programmes. This discussion should address ways to ensure that programmes are interesting, manageable and worthwhile.

ASSESSMENT OF HEALTH-RELATED LEARNING

- Towards the end of the unit of work, ask pupils questions such as the following:
  - How can you achieve progression in an exercise programme?
  - What does *overload* mean in relation to exercise?
  - Discuss with a partner what *specificity* means in relation to exercise and think of some examples to share with the class.
  - Why are balance, moderation and variety important when planning an exercise programme?
  - What helps people maintain an exercise programme?
  - What does *reversibility* mean in relation to exercise?
  - With a partner, weigh up the costs and benefits of following a three-month exercise programme.

HEALTH-RELATED LEARNING OUTCOMES: LESSONS 5 AND 6

ACTIVITY PROMOTION

- Assess their own qualities, skills, achievements and potential so that they can set personal goals that help them follow the activity recommendations for young people and develop a commitment to an active lifestyle.

- Explain constraints on being active and explore how to overcome them in order to access and sustain involvement in activity.

HEALTH-RELATED LEARNING ACTIVITIES

- In pairs, ask pupils to look over each other's activity journals in order to ascertain current activity levels and discuss personal activity goals. Is the partner meeting the age-specific recommendation for physical activity for health? If not, how can the partner increase his or her activity to work towards meeting the recommendation over time?

- During these lessons, give pupils a choice of activities, such as brisk walking, jogging, skipping, and toning or strengthening exercises (either with or without free dumbbells or elastics). Whilst pupils are involved in these activities, look over their activity journals and discuss their personal activity goals with them.

- During the final lesson, ask pupils to walk and jog with a partner while talking about barriers and constraints to being active and how to overcome them. This discussion should address what individuals and groups can do to address the barriers and constraints. Facilitate the sharing of responses with the class.

ASSESSMENT OF HEALTH-RELATED LEARNING

- Towards the end of the unit of work, ask pupils questions such as the following:
  - Set personal activity goals, taking into consideration your current activity levels, abilities and preferences.
  - What can you do in the next month to increase the amount of activity you do?

- Towards the end of the unit of work, involve pupils in active assessment tasks such as the following:
  - Walk and jog with a partner while talking about barriers and constraints to being active and how to overcome them.

- Walk and talk with a partner about how you might be able to help each other to be more active.

Short-term plans for health-related learning generally take the form of lesson plans with specific health-related learning outcomes that sit within units or blocks of work. The following example is a lesson plan for 15- and 16-year-olds that outlines learning outcomes for safety issues within an activity-based unit of work (focused on evaluating warm-ups), as well as learning activities to address the outcomes and suggested methods of assessing the learning.

HEALTH-RELATED LEARNING OUTCOMES

SAFETY ISSUES

- Evaluate warm-ups in terms of safety, effectiveness and relevance to the specific activity and take responsibility for their own safe and effective preparation for activity.

HEALTH-RELATED LEARNING ACTIVITIES

- Ask pupils to discuss in pairs or small groups what is involved in taking responsibility for one's own safe and effective preparation for activity.
- Ask pupils to work in small groups to design a warm-up for an aerobic activity announced by the teacher. Prompt them to consider issues associated with safety (occurs in an area free of hazards; increases intensity gradually), effectiveness (incorporates developmentally appropriate mobility exercises, aerobic activities and stretches) and relevance (relates to the activity to follow it in terms of the joints mobilised, the aerobic activities selected and the muscle groups stretched). Relevance can also be enhanced by making use of the equipment and area associated with the activity (e.g., for badminton, using a racket, a shuttlecock or lines on the court).
- Afterwards, ask the pupils in each group to lead another small group through their warm-up. The group being led then evaluates the warm-up by responding to the following questions:
  1. Was the area clear of potential hazards during the warm-up?
  2. Did the intensity of the warm-up build gradually?
  3. Did the warm-up include developmentally appropriate mobility exercises, aerobic activities and stretches?
  4. In what ways was the warm-up related to the activity to follow it?
  5. How might the warm-up be improved?
- Following the warm-up, involve pupils in the lesson activity.
- Towards the end of the lesson, ask pupils to perform a cool-down that involves low-intensity aerobic activities and static stretches of the major muscle groups used in the activity.

ASSESSMENT OF HEALTH-RELATED LEARNING

- What is involved in taking responsibility for your own safe and effective preparation for activity?
- What makes a warm-up safe?
- What makes a warm-up effective?
- What makes a warm-up relevant?
- Design and lead others through a warm-up for a specific activity.
- Observe a group's warm-up and then provide feedback on its safety, effectiveness and relevance.

This lesson can be facilitated by using the form titled Evaluating a Warm-Up in the web resource for this chapter.

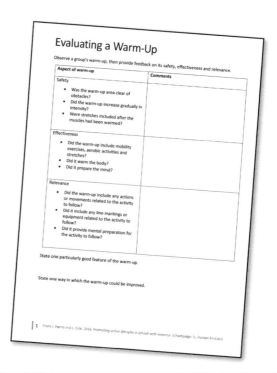

Summary

If you take a structured, progressive approach to children's learning about leading a healthy, active lifestyle, then you can engage them with this important aspect of the curriculum in way that is comprehensive, coherent and meaningful. This sort of approach needs to be evident at all stages of schooling and be accessible to every pupil.

One good way to start is to develop health-related learning plans that include relevant outcomes for successive age groups. The learning can then be organised, taught and assessed in multiple ways and can incorporate the monitoring of children's health, activity and fitness through methods that are developmentally appropriate and pedagogically desirable.

Glossary

accessibility—Full entitlement to the curriculum by all pupils; a responsibility of teachers.

active pedagogies—Teaching and learning approaches that increase pupils' level of activity during lessons.

affective outcome—Outcome related to feelings and attitudes (e.g., positive attitude toward physical education).

asthma—Long-term inflammatory disease of the airways characterised by episodes of wheezing, coughing, chest tightness and shortness of breath.

behavioural outcome—Outcome associated with actions (e.g., participating in a school sport club).

body composition—This refers to the proportions of muscle, fat, bone and water in the body.

body mass index (BMI)—Measure defined as body mass (in kilograms) divided by the square of height (in metres).

cardiovascular disease—Class of disease that affects the heart or blood vessels (e.g., angina, heart attack, stroke).

cardiovascular disease (CVD) risk profile—Prevalence of factors in an individual that are associated with disease affecting the heart or blood vessels (e.g., family history, sedentary lifestyle, overweight, obesity, high cholesterol, high blood pressure, stress).

cardiorespiratory fitness—Ability of the cardiorespiratory system (i.e., heart, blood vessels, lungs) to function efficiently and cope with the demands made on it.

chronic condition—Condition or disease that is persistent and long lasting (e.g., arthritis, asthma, cancer, diabetes, heart disease).

cognitive outcome—Outcome related to knowledge and understanding (e.g., knowing the social health benefits of being active).

criterion-referenced standards—Fixed set of predetermined criteria or written descriptions.

diabetes—Condition in which the amount of glucose (sugar) in the blood is too high either because the pancreas does not produce any or enough insulin or because the insulin produced does not work properly.

energy balance—Relationship between energy intake and energy expenditure.

energy expenditure—Amount of energy (i.e., number of calories) used in functions such as breathing, digestion and movement.

entitlement—Fundamental right, in this context the right of all children to access education.

FITT principle—Principle in which the acronym *FITT* refers to the frequency, intensity, time and type of physical activity and which is used to guide the development of activity and fitness training programmes to meet individual needs.

flexibility—Range of movement around a joint.

health—State characterized by a person's mental and/or physical condition; not merely by the absence of disease or infirmity but by complete physical, mental and social well-being; a resource for everyday life; a positive concept emphasising social and personal resources, as well as physical capacities.

health and fitness—Used to describe learning associated with health and fitness within curriculum physical education.

health-based physical education (HBPE)—Approach that involves learning to value and practice appropriate physical activities that enhance health and well-being.

health education—Planned opportunities to develop knowledge and life skills conducive to individual and community health.

health-related components of fitness—These are associated with health outcomes and include cardiorespiratory fitness, muscular strength and endurance, flexibility and body composition.

health-related exercise—Used to describe learning associated with health within curriculum physical education.

health-related fitness—Used to describe learning associated with health and fitness within curriculum physical education.

health-related learning—Learning associated with adopting a lifestyle conducive to good health.

hypokinetic—Associated with insufficient activity or with diminished motor function or power of movement.

inclusion—Approach that recognises a continuum of learning needs and involves planning and delivering lessons to meet those needs.

inclusion spectrum—Activity-centred approach to the inclusion of pupils with different abilities in physical activity.

integrity—Principle concerned with ensuring that all teaching, learning and assessment approaches and tasks are of equal worth and in no way tokenistic or patronising.

lean body mass—Body mass or weight excluding body fat.

morbidity—Incidence or prevalence of a disease.

motor fitness—This is associated with performance outcomes and is sometimes referred to as performance- or skill-related fitness; it includes agility, balance, coordination, power, reaction time and speed.

muscular strength and endurance—Ability of the musculoskeletal system (i.e., bones, muscles, joints, tendons, ligaments) to work against resistance over time.

norm-referenced standard—Standard involving comparison of an individual's score with that of a reference group (i.e., determining whether the individual did better or worse than others).

obesity—Medical condition in which excess body fat has accumulated to the extent that it may have a negative effect on health.

obesogenic environment—Environment that encourages people to eat unhealthily and not do enough exercise, thus contributing to obesity (e.g., places that encourage cars over walking, buildings with lifts and escalators prominently sited and stairs hidden away, public places dominated by shops selling calorie-dense foods).

overweight—Having more body fat than is optimally healthy.

performance-related (skill-related) components of fitness—These are associated with performance outcomes and include agility, balance, coordination, power, reaction time and speed; this type of fitness is sometimes referred to as motor fitness.

physical activity—Any bodily movement produced by skeletal muscle that results in energy expenditure above that of resting.

physical fitness—Set of attributes related to the ability to perform physical activity.

STEP model—Framework for facilitating all pupils' involvement in physical activity based on modifications made by teachers to one or more of four areas (space, task, equipment, people).

References

Chapter 1

American College of Sports Medicine (ACSM). (1988). Opinion statement on physical fitness in children and youth. *Medicine and Science in Sport and Exercise, 20*(4), 422–423.

American College of Sports Medicine (ACSM). (1991). *Guidelines for exercise testing and prescription* (4th ed.). Philadelphia: Lea & Febiger.

American College of Sports Medicine (ACSM). (1995). *ACSM's guidelines for exercise testing and prescription* (5th ed.). Baltimore: Williams & Wilkins.

Australian Curriculum and Reporting Authority. (2011). Australian curriculum. www.australiancurriculum.edu.au/

Biddle, S., & Asare, M. (2011). Physical activity and mental health in children and adolescents: A review of reviews. *British Journal of Sports Medicine,* 45(11), 886-895.

Brusseau, T.A., Kulinna, P.H., & Cothran, D.J. (2011). Health and physical activity content knowledge of Pima children. *Kinesiology, Sport Studies and Physical Education Faculty Publications, 64.* Brockport, NY: College at Brockport, State University of New York.

Burrows, L. (2008) 'Fit, fast, and skinny': New Zealand school pupils 'talk' about health. *Journal of Physical Education New Zealand, 41*(3), 26–36.

Burrows, L., & Wright, J. (2004). The good life: New Zealand children's perspectives on health and self. *Sport, Education and Society, 9*(2), 193–205.

Burrows, L., Wright, J., & Jungersen-Smith, J. (2002). 'Measure your belly': New Zealand children's constructions of health and fitness. *Journal of Teaching in Physical Education, 22*(1), 39–48.

Burrows, L., Wright, J., & McCormack, J. (2009). Dosing up on food and physical activity: New Zealand children's ideas about 'health'. *Health Education Journal, 68*(3), 157–169.

Cale, L., & Harris, J. (Eds.). (2005). *Exercise and young people: Issues, implications and initiatives.* Basingstoke: Palgrave Macmillan.

Cale, L., & Harris, J. (2006). School-based physical activity interventions—Effectiveness, trends, issues, implications and recommendations for practice. *Sport, Education and Society, 11*(4), 401–420.

Cale, L., & Harris, J. (2009). *Getting the buggers fit* (2nd ed.). London: Continuum.

Corbin, C.B., Pangrazi, R.P., & Welk, G.J. (1994). Toward an understanding of appropriate physical activity levels for youth. *Physical Activity and Fitness Research Digest, 1*(8), 1–7.

Currie, C., Gabhainn, S., Godeau, E., Roberts, C., Smith, R., Currie, D., . . . Barnekow, V. (Eds.). (2008). *Inequalities in young people's health: International report from the HBSC 2005/06 survey.* WHO Policy Series: Health Policy for Children and Adolescents, Issue 5. Copenhagen: WHO Regional Office for Europe.

De Meester, F., van Lenthe, J.J., Spittaels, H., Lien, N., & De Bourdeauhuij, I. (2009). Interventions for promoting physical activity among European teenagers: A systematic review. *International Journal of Behavioural Nutrition and Physical Activity, 6*(82), 1–11.

Demetriou, Y., & Honer, O. (2012). Physical activity interventions in the school setting: A systematic review. *Psychology of Sport and Exercise, 13,* 186–196.

Department for Education. (2013). *National curriculum in England: Physical education programmes of study.* www.gov.uk/government/publications/national-curriculum-in-england-physical-education-programmes-of-study

Department of Health. (2009). *Change4Life.* www.nhs.uk/Change4Life.

Department of Health; Department of Health, Social Sciences and Public Safety; Scottish Government, & Welsh Government. (2011). *Start active, stay active: A report on physical activity for health from the four home countries' chief medical officers.* www.gov.uk/government/publications/start-active-stay-active-a-report-on-physical-activity-from-the-four-home-countries-chief-medical-officers

Dixey, R., Sahota, P., Atwal, S., & Turner, A. (2001). 'Ha ha, you're fat, we're strong': A qualitative study of boys' and girls' perceptions of fatness, thinness, social pressures and health using focus groups. *Health Education, 101*(5), 206–216.

Dobbins, M., De Corby, K., Robeson, P., Husson, H., & Tirilis, D. (2009). School-based physical activity programs for promoting physical activity and fitness in children and adolescents aged 6 to 18. *Cochrane Database of Systematic Reviews*, 1.

Dobbins, M., Husson, H., De Corby, K., & La Rocca, R.L. (2013). School-based physical activity programs for promoting physical activity and fitness in children and adolescents aged 6 to 18. *Cochrane Database of Systematic Reviews*, 2.

Donnelly, J. E., Hillman, C. H., Castelli, D., Etnier, J. L., Lee, S., Tomporowski, P., Lambourne, K., & Szabo-Reed, A. N. (2016). Physical activity, fitness, cognitive function, and academic achievement in children: A systematic review. *Medicine and Science in Sports and Exercise, 48*(6), 1197-1222.

Fedewa, A.L., & Ahn, S. (2011). The effects of physical activity and physical fitness on children's achievement and cognitive outcomes. *Research Quarterly for Exercise and Sport, 82*(3), 521–535.

Gard, M., & Pluim, C. (2014). *Schools and public health: Past, present, future*. Plymouth, UK: Lexington Books.

Harris, J. (1993). Young people's perceptions of health, fitness and exercise. *British Journal of Physical Education Research Supplement, 13*, 5–9.

Harris, J. (1994) Young people's perceptions of health, fitness and exercise: Implications for the teaching of health-related exercise. *Physical Education Review, 17*(2), 143–151.

Harris, J., Cale, L., Duncombe, R., & Musson, H. (2016). Young people's knowledge and understanding of health, fitness and physical activity: Issues, divides and dilemmas. *Sport, Education and Society*. doi: 10.1080/13573322.2016.1228047

Health and Social Care Information Centre (HSCIC). (2008). *Health Survey for England—2007*. www.hscic.gov.uk/pubs/hse07healthylifestyles

Health and Social Care Information Centre (HSCIC). (2016). *Health Survey for England—2015*. www.gov.uk/government/statistics/health-survey-for-england-health-survey-for-england-2015

Health and Social Care Information Centre (HSCIC). (2015). *Statistics on obesity, physical activity and diet: England 2015*. www.gov.uk/government/statistics/statistics-on-obesity-physical-activity-and-diet-england-2015

Janssen, L., & LeBlanc, A.G. (2010). Systematic review of the health benefits of physical activity and fitness in school-aged children and youth. *International Journal of Behavioural Nutrition and Physical Activity, 7*, 7–40.

Keating, X.D., Harrison, L., Chen, L., Xiang, P., Lambdin, D., Dauenhauer, B., . . . Pinero, J.C. (2009). An analysis of research on student health-related fitness knowledge in K-16 physical education programs. *Journal of Teaching in Physical Education, 28*(3), 333–349.

Keeley, T.J.H., & Fox, K. (2009). The impact of physical activity and fitness on academic achievement and cognitive performance in children. *International Review of Sport and Exercise Psychology, 2*(2), 198–214.

Kirk, D., & Colquhoun, D. (1989). Healthism and physical education. *British Journal of Sociology of Education, 10*, 417–434.

Kriemler, S., Meyer, U., Martin, E., Van Sluijs, E.M.F., Andersen, L.B., & Martin, B.W. (2011). Effect of school-based interventions on physical activity and fitness in children and adolescents: A review of reviews and systematic update. *British Journal of Sports Medicine, 45*(11), 923–930.

Lee, J., & Macdonald, D. (2009). Rural young people and physical activity: Understanding participation through social theory. *Sociology of Health and Illness, 31*(3), 360–374.

Lee, J., & Macdonald, D. (2010). 'Are they just checking our obesity or what?' The healthism discourse and rural young women. *Sport, Education and Society, 15*(2), 203–219.

Merkle, D.G., & Treagust, D.F. (1993). Student knowledge of health and fitness concepts and its relation to locus of control. *School Science and Mathematics, 93*, 355–359.

Morrow, J., Jr., Scott, R., Martin, B., & Jackson, A.W. (2010). Reliability and validity of the Fitnessgram: Quality of teacher-collected health-related fitness surveillance data. *Research Quarterly for Exercise and Sport, 81*(Suppl. 3), S24–S30.

National Institute for Health and Care Excellence (NICE). (2008a). *Physical activity and children. Review 1: Descriptive epidemiology*. www.nice.org.uk/guidance/ph17/evidence/review-1-epidemiology-revised-july-2008-pdf-371243053

National Institute for Health and Care Excellence (NICE). (2008b). *Physical activity and the environment*. www.nice.org.uk/guidance/ph8

National Institute for Health and Care Excellence (NICE). (2009). *Promoting physical activity for children and young people*. www.nice.org.uk/guidance/ph17

National Institute for Health and Care Excellence (NICE). (2015). *Obesity in children and young people: Prevention and lifestyle weight management programmes*. Quality standard. Published: 23 July 2015. www.nice.org.uk/guidance/qs94/resources/obesity-in-children-and-young-people-prevention-and-lifestyle-weight-management-programmes-pdf-2098969040581

Organisation for Economic Co-operation and Development (OECD). (2013). *Health at a glance 2013: OECD indicators*. www.oecd-ilibrary.org/social-issues-migration-health/health-at-a-glance-2013_health_glance-2013-en

O'Shea, J.M., & Beausoleil, N. (2012). Breaking down 'healthism': Barriers to health and fitness as identified by immigrant youth in St. John's, NL, Canada. *Sport, Education and Society*, *17*(1), 97–112.

Physical Activity Guidelines Advisory Committee (2008). *Physical activity guidelines advisory committee report 2008*. Washington, DC: Department of Health and Human Services. https://health.gov/paguidelines/report/pdf/CommitteeReport.pdf

Placek, J., Griffin, L., Dodds, P., Raymond, C., Tremino, F., & James, A. (2001). Middle schools pupils' conceptions of fitness: The long road to a healthy lifestyle. *Journal of Teaching in Physical Education*, *20*, 314–323.

Plowman, S.A., Sterling, C.L., Corbin, C.B., Meredith, M.D., Welk, G.J., & Morrow, J.R. (2006). The history of Fitnessgram. *Journal of Physical Activity & Health*, *3*(2), S5–S20.

Powell, D., & Fitzpatrick, K. (2015). 'Getting fit basically just means, like, nonfat': Children's lessons in fitness and fatness. *Sport, Education and Society*, *20*(4), 463–484.

Public Health England. (2014a). *Everybody active, every day: An evidence-based approach to physical activity*. www.gov.uk/government/uploads/system/uploads/attachment_data/file/374914/Framework_13.pdf

Public Health England. (2014b). *Everybody active, every day: Implementation and evidence guide*. www.gov.uk/government/uploads/system/uploads/attachment_data/file/353385/Everybody_Active__Every_Day_Implementation__Evidence_Guide_CONSULTATION_VERSION.pdf

Public Health England. (2015). *Change4Life evidence review. Rapid evidence review on the effect of physical activity participation among children aged 5-11 years*. www.gov.uk/government/publications/change4life-evidence-review-on-physical-activity-in-children

Roth, M., & Stamatakis, E. (2010). Linking young people's knowledge of public health guidelines to physical activity levels in England. *Pediatric Exercise Sciences*, *22*, 467–476.

Scottish Government. (2016). *The Scottish Health Survey 2015*. www.gov.scot/Publications/2016/09/2764/downloads#res-1

Sport Northern Ireland. (2009). *Activ8*. www.activ8ni.net

Sport Northern Ireland (2016). *Young people and sport in Northern Ireland*. http://www.sportni.net/sportni/wp-content/uploads/2016/12/Young-People-and-Sport.pdf

Stensel, D.J., Gorely, T., & Biddle, S.J.H. (2008). Youth health outcomes. In A.L. Smith & S.J.H. Biddle (Eds.), *Youth physical activity and sedentary behaviour: Challenges and solutions* (pp. 31–57). Champaign, IL: Human Kinetics.

Stewart, S., & Mitchell, M. (2003). Instructional variables and student knowledge and conceptions of fitness. *Journal of Teaching in Physical Education*, *22*(5), 533–551.

St. Leger, L. (2004). What's the place of schools in promoting health? Are we too optimistic? *Health Promotion International*, *19*(4), 405–408.

Stone, E.J., McKenzie, T.L., Welk, G.J., & Booth, M.L. (1998). Effects of physical activity interventions in youth: Review and synthesis. *American Journal of Preventive Medicine*, *15*(4), 298–315.

Telema, R. (2009). Tracking of physical activity from childhood to adulthood: a review. *Obesity Facts*, *2*, 187-195.

Thomas, K.T. (2004). Riding to the rescue while holding on by a thread: Physical activity in the schools. *Quest*, *56*(1), 150–170.

Twisk, J.W.R., Kemper, H.C.G., & Van Mechelen, W. (2000). Tracking of activity and fitness and the relationship with cardiovascular disease risk factors. *Medicine and Science in Sports and Exercise*, *32*(8), 1455–1461.

Twisk, J.W.R., Kemper, H.C.G., & Van Mechelen, W. (2002). Prediction of cardiovascular disease risk factors in later life by physical activity and fitness in youth: General comments and conclusions. *International Journal of Sports Science*, *23*(Suppl.), S440–S450.

Tymms, P.B., Curtis, S.E., Routen, A.C., Thomson, K.H., Bolden, D.S., Bock, S., . . . Kasim, A.S. (2016). Clustered randomised controlled trial of two education interventions designed to increase physical activity and well-being of secondary school students: The MOVE Project. *British Medical Journal Open*, *6*(1). doi:10.1135/bmjopen-2015-009318

United Nations Children's Fund (UNICEF). (2007). *Child poverty in perspective: An overview of child well-being in rich countries*. Innocenti Report Card 7. Florence: UNICEF Innocenti Research Centre.

United Nations Children's Fund (UNICEF). (2013). *Child well-being in rich countries: A comparative review*. Innocenti Report Card 11. Florence: UNICEF Office of Research.

United Nations Children's Fund (UNICEF). (2016). *Fairness for children: A league table of inequality in child well-being in rich countries*. Innocenti Report Card 13. Florence: UNICEF Office of Research.

van Sluijs, E.M.F., McMinn, A.M., & Griffin, S.J. (2007). Effectiveness of interventions to promote physical activity in children and adolescents: Systematic review of controlled trials. *British Medical Journal, 335*, 703.

Welsh Government. (2017). *Welsh Health Survey 2016*. http://gov.wales/statistics-and-research/welsh-health-survey/?lang=en

World Health Organisation (WHO). (2005). *Atlas: Child and adolescent health mental resources: Global concerns: Implications for the future*. Geneva: WHO Press. www.who.int/mental_health/resources/Child_ado_atlas.pdf

World Health Organisation (WHO). (2008). *School policy framework: Implementation of the WHO global strategy on diet, physical activity and health*. Geneva: WHO Press. www.who.int/dietphysicalactivity/schools/en/

World Health Organisation (WHO). (2010). *Global recommendations on physical activity for health*. Geneva: WHO Press. www.who.int/dietphysicalactivity/factsheet_recommendations/en/

World Health Organisation (WHO). (2016). *Report of the commission on ending childhood obesity*. Geneva: WHO Press. http://apps.who.int/iris/bitstream/10665/204176/1/9789241510066_eng.pdf

Chapter 2

British Heart Foundation. (1999a). *The active school. Section 4: Active breaktimes and lunchtimes*. Loughborough: Author.

British Heart Foundation. (1999b). *The active school. Section 3: PE & physical activity across the curriculum*. Loughborough: Author.

Cale, L. (1997). Promoting physical activity through the active school. *British Journal of Physical Education, 28*(1), 19–21.

Cale, L., & Harris, J. (2009). *Getting the buggers fit* (2nd ed.). London: Continuum.

Clemes, S., Barber, S.E., Bingham, D.D., Ridgers, N.D., Fletcher, E., Pearson, N., . . . Dunstan, D.W. (2015). Reducing children's classroom sitting time using sit-to-stand desks: Findings from pilot studies in UK and Australian primary schools. *Journal of Public Health, 38*(3), 526–533.

Department for Education and Employment. (1999). *National healthy school standard: Guidance*. London: Department for Education and Employment.

Department of Health. (2005). *National healthy school status: A guide for schools*. London: Department of Health Publications.

Donnelly, J.E. (2011). Classroom-based activity, cognition and academic achievement. *Preventive Medicine, 52*, S36–S42.

Fox, K. (1996). Physical activity promotion and the active school. In N. Armstrong (Ed.), *New directions in physical education* (pp. 94–109). London: Cassell Education.

Gustafson, S.L., & Rhodes, R.E. (2006). Parental correlates of physical activity in children and early adolescents. *Sports Medicine, 36*(1), 79–97.

Jago, R., Fox, K.R., Page, A.S., Brockman, R., & Thompson, J.L. (2010). Parent and child physical activity and sedentary time: Do active parents foster active children? *BMC Public Health, 10*, 194.

Lowden, K., Powney, J., Davidson, J., & James, C. (2001). *The Class Moves! pilot in Scotland and Wales*. Glasgow: SCRE Centre, University of Glasgow.

Lubans, D.R., Morgan, P.J., & Tudor-Locke, C. (2009). A systematic review of studies using pedometers to promote physical activity among youth. *Preventive Medicine, 48*(4), 307–315.

McMullen, J., Ni Chroinin, D., Tammelin, T., Pogorzelska, M., & Van der Mars, H. (2015). International approaches to whole-of-school physical activity promotion. *Quest, 67*(4), 384–399.

Scottish Government. (2008). *Schools (health promotion and nutrition) Scotland act: Health promotion guidance for local authorities and schools*. www.gov.scot/Publications/2008/05/08160456/0

Scottish Health Promoting Schools Unit. (2004). *Being well—Doing well: A framework for health promoting schools in Scotland*. Learning and Teaching Scotland.

Stathi, A., Nordin, S., & Riddoch, C. (2006). *Evaluation of the 'Schools on the Move' project on behalf of the Youth Sport Trust, Department for Education and Skills and the Department of Health*. London: London Sport Institute, Middlesex University.

Stewart-Brown, S. (2006). *What is the evidence on school health promotion in improving health or preventing disease and, specifically, what is the effectiveness of the health promoting schools approach?* Copenhagen: WHO Regional Office for Europe (Health Evidence Network report).

Welsh Assembly Government. (2009). *Indicators for the Welsh Network of Healthy School Schemes National Quality Award*. Cardiff: Author.

World Health Organisation. (2012). *Health education: Theoretical concepts, effective strategies and core competencies*. Cairo: WHO Regional Office for the Eastern Mediterranean.

Chapter 3

Armour, K., & Harris, J. (2013). Making the case for developing new 'PE-for-health' pedagogies. *Quest, 65*(2), 201–219.

Association for Young People's Health. (2017). *Key data on adolescence 2017* (11th ed.). www.youngpeopleshealth.org.uk/key-data-on-adolescence

Bailey, R., Armour, K., Kirk, D., Jess, M., Pickup, I., Sandford, R., & BERA Physical Education and Sport Pedagogy Special Interest Group. (2009). The educational benefits claimed for physical education and school sport: An academic review. *Research Papers in Education*, *24*(1), 1–27.

Burrows, L., Wright, J., & McCormack, J. (2009). Dosing up on food and physical activity: New Zealand children's ideas about 'health'. *Health Education Journal*, *68*(3), 157–169.

Cale, L., Casey, A., & Harris, J. (2016). An advocacy paper for physical education and school sport. *Physical Education Matters*, *11*(1), 18–19.

Cale, L., & Harris, J. (2006). School-based physical activity interventions: Effectiveness, trends, issues, implications and recommendations for practice. *Sport, Education and Society*, *11*(4), 401–420.

Council for the Curriculum, Examinations and Assessment. (2014). *Statutory requirements for physical education*. http://ccea.org.uk/curriculum/key_stage_1_2/areas_learning/physical_education

Department for Education. (2013). *Statutory guidance: National curriculum in England: Physical education programmes of study*. www.gov.uk/government/publications/national-curriculum-in-england-physical-education-programmes-of-study

Donnelly, J. E., Hillman, C. H., Castelli, D., Etnier, J. L., Lee, S., Tomporowski, P., Lambourne, K., & Szabo-Reed, A. N. (2016). Physical activity, fitness, cognitive function, and academic achievement in children: A systematic review. *Medicine and Science in Sports and Exercise*, *48*(6), 1197-1222.

Education Scotland (2017). *Benchmarks physical education*. https://education.gov.scot/improvement/Documents/HWBPhysicalEducationBenchmarksPDF.pdf

Fedewa, A.L., & Ahn, S. (2011). The effects of physical activity and physical fitness on children's achievement and cognitive outcomes. *Research Quarterly for Exercise and Sport*, *82*(3), 521–535.

Future Foundation. (2015). *The class of 2035: Promoting a brighter and more active future for the youth of tomorrow*. London: Author.

Haarens, L., Kirk, D., Cardon, G., & de Bourdeaudhuij, I. (2011). Toward the development of a pedagogical model for health-based physical education. *Quest*, *63*, 321–338.

Harris, J. (2000). *Health-related exercise in the national curriculum: Key stages 1 to 4*. Leeds: Human Kinetics.

Harris, J. (2009). Health-related exercise and physical education. In R. Bailey & D. Kirk (Eds.), *The Routledge physical education reader* (pp. 83–101). Oxon: Routledge.

Harris, J. (2015). afPE's position on health. *Physical Education Matters*, *10*(3), 87–90.

Harris, J., & Leggett, G. (2015a). Influences on the expression of health within physical education curricula in secondary schools in England and Wales. *Sport, Education and Society*, *20*(7), 908–923.

Harris, J., & Leggett, G. (2015b). Testing, training and tensions: The expression of health within physical education curricula in secondary schools in England and Wales. *Sport, Education and Society*, *20*(4), 423–441.

Keeley, T.J.H., & Fox, K. (2009). The impact of physical activity and fitness on academic achievement and cognitive performance in children. *International Review of Sport and Exercise Psychology*, *2*(2), 198–214.

Shephard, R.J., & Trudeau, F. (2000). The legacy of physical education: Influences on adult lifestyle. *Pediatric Exercise Science*, *12*, 34–50.

Welsh Assembly Government. (2008). *Physical education in the national curriculum for Wales*. http://learning.gov.wales/docs/learningwales/publications/130425-physical-education-inthe-national-curriculum-en.pdf

Chapter 4

Evans, J., Rich, E., Allwood, R., & Davies, B. (2007). Being 'able' in a performative culture. In: Wellard, I. (Ed.). *Rethinking Gender and Youth Sport*. London: Routledge, pp. 51-67.

Falconer, C.L., associated with Park, M.H., Croker, H., Skow, A., Black, J., Saxena, S., . . . Kinra, S. (2014). The benefits and harms of providing parents with weight feedback as part of the National Child Measurement Programme: A prospective cohort study. BioMed Central (BMC) Public Health, *14*, 549. doi: 10.1186/1471-2458-14-549

Health and Social Care Information Centre. (2015). National Child Measurement Programme: England, 2014/15 school year. Leeds: Author.

Lupton, D. (2014). Apps as artefacts: Towards a critical perspective on mobile health and medical apps. *Societies*, *4*, 606–622.

Public Health Wales. (2015). Child Measurement Programme for Wales 2013/2014. Cardiff: Public Health Wales NHS Trust.

United Nations Children's Fund (UNICEF). (2007) *Child poverty in perspective: An overview of child well-being in rich countries*. Innocenti Report Card 7. Florence: UNICEF Innocenti Research Centre.

United Nations Children's Fund (UNICEF). (2013). *Child well-being in rich countries: A comparative review*. Innocenti Report Card 11. Florence: UNICEF Office of Research.

World Health Organisation. (1948). Preamble to the Constitution of WHO as adopted by the International Health Conference, New York, 19 June - 22 July 1946; signed on 22 July 1946 by the representatives of 61 States (Official Records of WHO, no. 2, p. 100) and entered into force on 7 April 1948.

World Health Organisation (1986). The Ottawa Charter for Health Promotion. First International Conference on Health Promotion, Ottawa, 21 November 1986.

World Health Organisation. (2005). *Atlas: Child and adolescent mental health resources: Global concerns: Implications for the future*. Geneva: WHO Press. www.who.int/mental_health/resources/Child_ado_atlas.pdf.

Chapter 5

Biddle, S.J.H., Gorely, T., Pearson, N., & Bull, F.C. (2011) An assessment of self-reported physical activity instruments in young people for population surveillance: Project ALPHA. *International Journal of Behavioral Nutrition and Physical Activity*, *8*(1), 1–9.

Cale, L., & Harris, J. (2009). *Getting the buggers fit* (2nd ed.). London: Continuum.

Dollman, J., Okely, A.D., Hardy, L., Timperio, A., Salmon, J., & Hills, P. (2009). A hitchhiker's guide to assessing young people's physical activity: Deciding what method to use. *Journal of Science and Medicine in Sport*, *12*, 518–525.

Kohl, H.W., Fulton, J.E. & Caspersen, C.J. (2000). Assessment of physical activity among children and adolescents: a review and synthesis. *Preventive Medicine*, *31*(2), S54-S76.

Loprinzi, P.D., & Cardinal, B.J. (2011). Measuring children's physical activity and sedentary behaviour. *Journal of Exercise Science and Fitness*, *9*(1), 15–23.

Sallis, J.F., & Saelens, B.E. (2000). Assessment of physical activity by self-report: status, limitations, and future directions. *Research Quarterly for Exercise and Sport*, *71*(sup2), 1-14.

Salmon J., Tremblay, M.S., Marshall, S.J., & Hume, C. (2011). Health risks, correlates, and interventions to reduce sedentary behavior in young people. *American Journal of Preventive Medicine*, *41*, 197–206.

Sanders, J.P., Loveday, A., Pearson, N., Edwardson C., Yates, T., Biddle, S.J, Esliger, D.W. (2016). Devices for self-monitoring sedentary time or physical activity: A scoping review. *Journal of Medical Internet Research*, *18*(5), 90. doi: 10.2196/jmir.5373.

Trost, S.G. (2007). Measurement of physical activity in children and adolescents. *American Journal of Lifestyle Medicine*, *1*, 299–314.

Wilmot, E.G., Edwardson, C.L., Achana, F.A., Davies, M.J., Gorely, T., Gray, L.J., . . . Biddle, S.J.H. (2012). Sedentary time in adults and the association with diabetes, cardiovascular disease and death: Systematic review and meta-analysis. *Diabetologia*, *55*, 2895–2905.

Chapter 6

Association for Physical Education (afPE). (2016). *Safe practice in physical education*. Leeds: Coachwise.

Association for Physical Education (afPE). (2015a, October). *Health position paper*. www.afpe.org.uk/physical-education/wp-content/uploads/afPE_Health_Position_Paper_Web_Version2015.pdf

Association for Physical Education (afPE). (2015b). To fitness test—Or not? Association for Physical Education response to Generation Inactive. *Physical Education Matters*, *10*(3), 11.

Cale, L. (2016). Teaching about healthy active lifestyles. In C.D. Ennis (Ed), *The handbook of physical education* (pp. 399–411). London: Routledge.

Cale, L., & Harris, J. (Eds.). (2005). *Exercise and young people: Issues, implications and initiatives*. Basingstoke: Palgrave Macmillan.

Cale, L., & Harris, J. (2009a). Fitness testing in physical education—A misdirected effort in promoting healthy lifestyles and physical activity? *Physical Education and Sport Pedagogy*, *14*(1), 89–108.

Cale, L., & Harris, J. (2009b). *Getting the buggers fit* (2nd ed.). London: Continuum.

Cale, L., Harris, J., & Chen, M.H. (2014). Monitoring health, activity and fitness in physical education: Its current and future state of health. *Sport Education and Society*, *19*(4), 376–397.

Caspersen, C.J., Powell, K.E., & Christenson, G.M. (1985). Physical activity, exercise and physical fitness: Definitions and distinctions for health-related research. *Public Health Reports*, *100*, 126–130.

Cohen, D., Voss, C., & Sandercock, R.H. (2014). Fitness testing for children: Let's mount the zebra! *Journal of Physical Activity and Health*, *12*(5), 597–603.

Cooper Institute. (2017). *Fitnessgram administration manual: The journey to MyHealthyZone* (5th ed.). Champaign, IL: Human Kinetics.

Evans, J. (2007). Health education or weight management in schools? *Cardiometabolic Risk and Weight Management*, *2*(2), 12–16.

Evans, J., Rich, E., Davies, B., & Allwood, R. (2008). *Education, disordered eating and obesity discourse: Fat fabrications*. Oxon: Routledge.

Keating, X.D. (2003). The current often implemented fitness tests in physical education programs: Problems and future directions. *Quest*, *55*, 141–160.

Lloyd, M., Colley, R., & Tremblay, M.S. (2010). Advancing the debate on fitness testing for children:

Perhaps we're riding the wrong animal. *Pediatric Exercise Science, 22*, 176–182.

Naughton, G.A., Carlson, J.S., & Greene, D.A. (2006). A challenge to fitness testing in primary schools. *Journal of Science and Medicine in Sport, 9*, 40–45.

Pate, R.R. (1988). The evolving definition of physical fitness. *Quest, 40*, 174–179.

Rice, C. (2007). Becoming 'the fat girl': Acquisition of an unfit identity. *Women's Studies International Forum, 30*, 158–174.

Rowland, T.W. (2007). Fitness testing in schools: Once more around the track. *Pediatric Exercise Science, 19*, 113–114.

Silverman, S., Keating, X.D., & Phillips, S.R. (2008). A lasting impression: A pedagogical perspective on youth fitness testing. *Measurement in Physical Education, 12*, 146–166.

Chapter 7

Alfrey, L., Cale, L., & Webb, L. (2012). Physical education teachers' continuing professional development in health-related exercise. *Physical Education and Sport Pedagogy, 17*(5), 477–491.

Armour, K., & Harris, J. (2013). Making the case for developing new PE-for-health pedagogies. *Quest, 65*(2), 201–219.

Association for Physical Education (afPE). (2016). *Safe practice in physical education, school sport and physical activity*. Leeds: Coachwise.

Asthma UK. (2016a). *Exercise and activities*. www.asthma.org.uk/advice/living-with-asthma/exercise-and-activities/.

Asthma UK. (2016b). *What is asthma?* www.asthma.org.uk/advice/understanding-asthma/what-is-asthma/.

British Heart Foundation (BHF). (2011). *Physical activity for all: Physical activity for children and young people with medical conditions* [Course manual]. Loughborough: Loughborough University, BHF National Centre for Physical Activity and Health.

British Lung Foundation. (2016). *Asthma in children*. www.blf.org.uk/support-for-you/asthma/children.

Cale, L. (2011). *The promotion of healthy, active lifestyles through physical education: Challenges and opportunities*. Presentation and paper in the proceedings of the AIESEP World Congress, La Coruna, Spain, October 2010.

Cale, L., & Harris, J. (2009). *Getting the buggers fit* (2nd ed.). London: Continuum.

Cale, L., & Harris, J. (2013). 'Every child (of every size) matters' in physical education! Physical education's role in childhood obesity. *Sport, Education and Society, 18*(4), 433–452.

Department for Education. (2015). *Supporting pupils at school with medical conditions: Statutory guidance for governing bodies of maintained schools and proprietors of academies in England*. London: Author.

Department of Health. (2007). *Obesity guidance for healthy schools co-ordinators and their partners*. London: Author.

Diabetes UK. (2014). *Type 1 diabetes at school: School pack*. www.diabetes.org.uk/Guide-to-diabetes/Schools/Diabetes-in-schools-resources/.

Diabetes UK. (2015). *Facts and stats*. www.diabetes.org.uk/Documents/Position%20statements/Facts%20and%20stats%20June%202015.pdf.

Diabetes UK. (2016). *Diabetes: The basics*. www.diabetes.org.uk/Guide-to-diabetes/What-is-diabetes/.

Elbourn, J., & James, A. (2013). *Fitness room activities for secondary schools: A guide to promoting effective learning about healthy active lifestyles*. Leeds: Coachwise.

Evans, J. (2007). Health education or weight management in schools? *Cardiometabolic Risk and Weight Management, 2*(2), 12–16.

Fitzgerald, H. (2011). Disabling experiences of physical education and youth sport. In K. Armour (Ed.), *Sport pedagogy. An introduction for teaching and coaching* (pp. 153–164). Englewood Cliffs, NJ: Prentice Hall.

Fitzgerald, H. (2012). Drawing on disabled students' experiences of physical education and stakeholder responses. *Sport, Education and Society, 17*(4), 443–462.

Fox, K., & Harris, J. (2003). Promoting physical activity through schools. In J. McKenna, & C. Riddoch (Eds.), *Perspectives on Health and Exercise* (pp. 181–201). Basingstoke: Palgrave Macmillan.

Global Asthma Network. (2014). *The global asthma report 2014*. Auckland: Author.

Green, K. (2004). Physical education, lifelong participation and 'the couch potato' society. *Physical Education and Sport Pedagogy, 9*(1), 73–86.

Green, K. (2009). Exploring the everyday 'philosophies' of physical education teachers from a sociological perspective. In R. Bailey & D. Kirk (Eds.), *The Routledge physical education reader* (pp. 183–206). London: Routledge Taylor & Francis.

Haerens, L., Kirk, D., Cardon, G., & De Bourdeaudhuij, I. (2011). Toward the development of a pedagogical model for health-based physical education. *Quest, 63*, 321–338.

Harris, J. (2000). *Health-related exercise in the national curriculum: Key stages 1 to 4*. Champaign, IL: Human Kinetics.

Harris, J., & Leggett, G. (2015a). Influences on the expression of health within physical education curricula in secondary schools in England and Wales. *Sport, Education and Society*, *20*(7), 908–923.

Harris, J., & Leggett, G. (2015b). Testing, training and tensions: The expression of health within physical education curricula in secondary schools in England and Wales. *Sport, Education and Society*, *20*(3–4), 423–441.

Health and Social Care Information Centre. (2015a). *Health survey for England, 2014*. http://content.digital.nhs.uk/catalogue/PUB19295/HSE2014-Sum-bklet.pdf

Health and Social Care Information Centre. (2015b). *Statistics on obesity, physical activity and diet: England 2015*. http://content.digital.nhs.uk/catalogue/PUB16988/obes-phys-acti-diet-eng-2015.pdf

HM Government. (2016). *Childhood obesity: A plan for action*. www.gov.uk/government/publications/childhood-obesity-a-plan-for-action

Kirk, D. (2010). Four relational issues and the bigger picture. In D. Kirk (Ed.), *Physical Education Futures* (pp. 97–120). Oxon: Routledge.

MacPhail, A., & Halbert, J. (2005). The implementation of the revised physical education syllabus in Ireland: Circumstances, rewards and costs. *European Physical Education Review*, *1*(3), 287–308.

National Institute for Clinical Excellence (NICE). (2006). *Obesity: Guidance on the prevention, identification, assessment and management of overweight and obesity in adults and children: Reference guide for local authorities, schools and early years providers, workplaces and the public*. London: Author.

National Institute for Health and Care Excellence (NICE). (2015). *Obesity: Prevention and lifestyle weight management in children and young people* [NICE quality standard 94]. www.nice.org.uk/qs94.

Puhse, U., Barker, D., Brettschneider, W.-D., Feldmeth, A.K., Gerlach, E., Mccuaig, L.A., . . . Gerber, M. (2011). International approaches to health-oriented physical education: Local health debates and differing conceptions of health. *International Journal of Physical Education*, *3*, 2–15.

Stevenson, P. (2009). The pedagogy of inclusive youth sport: working towards real solutions. In H. Fitzgerald (Ed.), *Disability and youth sport* (pp. 119–131). London: Routledge.

Tannehill, D. (2012). Physical education for all: The impact of standards and curriculum on student choice. In S. Dagkas & K. Armour (Eds.), *Inclusion and exclusion through sport* (pp. 233–245). London: Routledge.

Vickerman, P. (2010). Inclusive teaching and learning. In R. Bailey (Ed.), *Physical education for learning: A guide for secondary schools* (pp. 197–207). London: Continuum.

World Health Organisation. (2016). *Report of the commission on ending childhood obesity*. Geneva: WHO Press.

Chapter 8

Association for Physical Education (afPE). (2015). To fitness test—Or not? Association for Physical Education response to Generation Inactive. *Physical Education Matters*, *10*(3), 11.

Cale, L. (2016). Teaching about healthy active lifestyles. In C.D. Ennis (Ed.) *The handbook of physical education* (pp. 399–411). London: Routledge.

Cale, L., & Harris, J. (2009a). Fitness testing in physical education—A misdirected effort in promoting healthy lifestyles and physical activity? *Physical Education and Sport Pedagogy*, *14*(1), 89–108.

Cale, L., & Harris, J. (2009b). *Getting the buggers fit* (2nd ed.). London: Continuum.

Cale, L., Harris, J., & Chen, M.H. (2014). Monitoring health, activity and fitness in physical education: Its current and future state of health. *Sport Education and Society*, *19*(4), 376–397.

Lloyd, M., Colley, R., & Tremblay, M.S. (2010). Advancing the debate on fitness testing for children: Perhaps we're riding the wrong animal. *Pediatric Exercise Science*, *22*, 176–182.

Personal, Social, Health and Economic Education (PSHE) Association. (2014). PSHE education programme of study (Key stages 1–4). https://sip.derby.gov.uk/media/schoolsinformationportal/contentassets/documents/healthyschoolsprogramme/1pshe/PSHE%20Programmes%20of%20study%202014%20-%20KS%201-4.pdf

Rowland, T.W. (2007). Fitness testing in schools: Once more around the track. *Pediatric Exercise Science*, *19*, 113–114.

Silverman, S., Keating, X.D., & Phillips, S.R. (2008). A lasting impression: A pedagogical perspective on youth fitness testing. *Measurement in Physical Education*, *12*, 146–166.

Chapter 9

Cale, L. (2016). Teaching about healthy active lifestyles. In C.D. Ennis (Ed.), *The handbook of physical education* (pp. 399–411). London: Routledge.

Cale, L., & Harris, J. (2009a). Fitness testing in physical education—A misdirected effort in promoting healthy lifestyles and physical activity? *Physical Education and Sport Pedagogy*, *14*(1), 89–108.

Cale, L., & Harris, J. (2009b). *Getting the buggers fit* (2nd ed.). London: Continuum.

Cale, L., Harris, J., & Chen, M.H. (2014). Monitoring health, activity and fitness in physical education: Its current and future state of health. *Sport Education and Society*, *19*(4), 376–397.

Lloyd, M., Colley, R., & Tremblay, M.S. (2010). Advancing the debate on fitness testing for children: Perhaps we're riding the wrong animal. *Pediatric Exercise Science*, *22*, 176–182.

Personal, Social, Health and Economic Education (PSHE) Association. (2014). PSHE education programme of study (Key stages 1–4). https://sip.derby.gov.uk/media/schoolsinformationportal/contentassets/documents/healthyschoolsprogramme/1pshe/PSHE%20Programmes%20of%20study%202014%20-%20KS%201-4.pdf

Rowland, T.W. (2007). Fitness testing in schools: Once more around the track. *Pediatric Exercise Science*, *19*, 113–114.

Silverman, S., Keating, X.D., & Phillips, S.R. (2008). A lasting impression: A pedagogical perspective on youth fitness testing. *Measurement in Physical Education*, *12*, 146–166.

Chapter 10

Association for Physical Education (afPE). (2015a). *Health position paper*. www.afpe.org.uk/physical-education/wp-content/uploads/afPE_Health_Position_Paper_Web_Version2015.pdf

Association for Physical Education (afPE). (2015b). To fitness test—Or not? Association for Physical Education response to Generation Inactive. *Physical Education Matters*, *10*(3), 11.

Biddle, S.J.H., Gorely, T., Pearson, N., & Bull, F.C. (2011). An assessment of self-reported physical activity instruments in young people for population surveillance: Project ALPHA. *International Journal of Behavioral Nutrition and Physical Activity*, *8*(1), 1–9.

Cale, L. (2016). Teaching about healthy active lifestyles. In C.D. Ennis (Ed.), *The Handbook of Physical Education* (pp. 399–411). London: Routledge.

Cale, L., & Harris, J. (2009a). Fitness testing in physical education—A misdirected effort in promoting healthy lifestyles and physical activity? *Physical Education and Sport Pedagogy*, *14*(1), 89–108.

Cale, L., & Harris, J. (2009b). *Getting the buggers fit* (2nd ed.). London: Continuum.

Cale, L., Harris, J., & Chen, M.H. (2014). Monitoring health, activity and fitness in physical education: Its current and future state of health. *Sport Education and Society*, *19*(4), 376–397.

Lloyd, M., Colley, R., & Tremblay, M.S. (2010). Advancing the debate on fitness testing for children: Perhaps we're riding the wrong animal. *Pediatric Exercise Science*, *22*, 176–182.

PSHE Association. (2014). *PSHE education programme of study (Key stages 1–4)*. https://sip.derby.gov.uk/media/schoolsinformationportal/contentassets/documents/healthyschoolsprogramme/1pshe/PSHE%20Programmes%20of%20study%202014%20-%20KS%201-4.pdf

Rowland, T.W. (2007). Fitness testing in schools: Once more around the track. *Pediatric Exercise Science*, *19*, 113–114.

Silverman, S., Keating, X.D., & Phillips, S.R. (2008). A lasting impression: A pedagogical perspective on youth fitness testing. *Measurement in Physical Education*, *12*, 146–166.

Trost, S.G. (2007). Measurement of physical activity in children and adolescents. *American Journal of Lifestyle Medicine*, *1*, 299–314.

Chapter 11

Association for Physical Education (afPE). (2015a). *Health position paper*. www.afpe.org.uk/physical-education/wp-content/uploads/afPE_Health_Position_Paper_Web_Version2015.pdf

Association for Physical Education (afPE). (2015b). To fitness test—Or not? Association for Physical Education response to Generation Inactive. *Physical Education Matters*, *10*(3), *11*.

Biddle, S.J.H., Gorely, T., Pearson, N., & Bull, F.C. (2011). An assessment of self-reported physical activity instruments in young people for population surveillance: Project ALPHA. *International Journal of Behavioral Nutrition and Physical Activity*, *8*(1), 1–9.

Cale, L. (2016). Teaching about healthy active lifestyles. In C.D. Ennis (Ed.), *The Handbook of Physical Education* (pp. 399–411). London: Routledge.

Cale, L., & Harris, J. (2009a). Fitness testing in physical education—A misdirected effort in promoting healthy lifestyles and physical activity? *Physical Education and Sport Pedagogy*, *14*(1), 89–108.

Cale, L., & Harris, J. (2009b). *Getting the buggers fit* (2nd ed.). London: Continuum.

Cale, L., Harris, J., & Chen, M.H. (2014). Monitoring health, activity and fitness in physical education: Its current and future state of health. *Sport Education and Society*, *19*(4), 376–397.

Lloyd, M., Colley, R., & Tremblay, M.S. (2010). Advancing the debate on fitness testing for children: Perhaps we're riding the wrong animal. *Pediatric Exercise Science*, *22*, 176–182.

PSHE Association. (2014). *PSHE education programme of study (Key stages 1–4)*. https://sip.derby.gov.uk/media/schoolsinformationportal/contentassets/documents/healthyschoolsprogramme/1pshe/

PSHE%20Programmes%20of%20study%20 2014%20-%20KS%201-4.pdf

Rowland, T.W. (2007) Fitness testing in schools: Once more around the track. *Pediatric Exercise Science, 19*, 113–114.

Silverman, S., Keating, X.D., & Phillips, S.R. (2008). A lasting impression: A pedagogical perspective on youth fitness testing. *Measurement in Physical Education, 12*, 146–166.

Trost, S.G. (2007). Measurement of physical activity in children and adolescents. *American Journal of Lifestyle Medicine, 1*, 299–314.

Index

Note: The italicized *f* and *t* following page numbers refer to figures and tables, respectively.

About the Authors

Jo Harris, PhD, is director of teacher education and a reader in physical education and sport pedagogy in the School of Sport, Exercise and Health Sciences at Loughborough University in Loughborough, England. She has 12 years of teaching experience and 29 years of teacher training experience, and she was honoured in 2015 as a principal fellow of the Higher Education Academy for her significant and sustained contribution to excellence and leadership in the field. Harris has received many other awards for her teaching and contributions to the profession. She previously served as both vice president and president of the Physical Education Association of the United Kingdom, and she has authored resources and books for teachers and teacher educators. In her leisure time, she enjoys travelling, reading and recreational exercise.

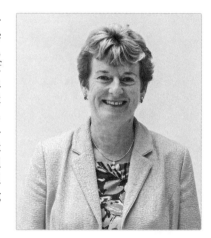

Lorraine Cale, PhD, is associate dean and a professor in physical education and sport pedagogy in the School of Sport, Exercise and Health Sciences at Loughborough University. She has worked in the areas of physical education and teacher education and been actively engaged in research on the promotion of physical activity and healthy lifestyles in schools, both within and beyond the curriculum, for many years. Cale has been published in academic and professional journals and has presented at numerous national and international conferences. She has also edited or authored three other books and numerous book chapters, and she has produced resources and training courses for teachers. Cale has twice been an elected member of the executive committee for the Association for Physical Education. She enjoys jogging, skiing, theatre and learning French.

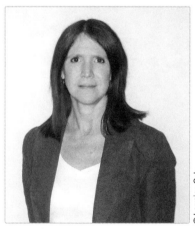

© Lorraine Cale

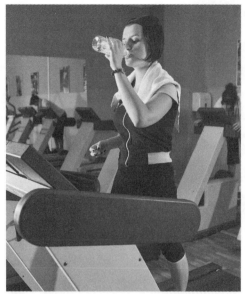
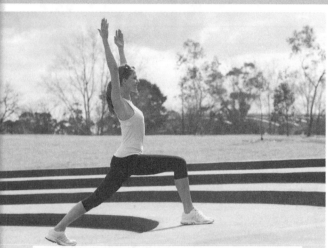
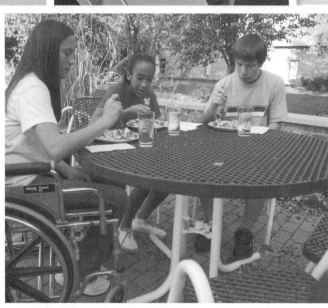
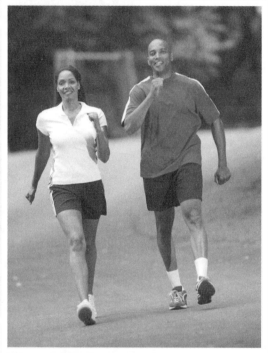
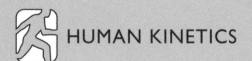